recipes for your
perfectly imperfect life

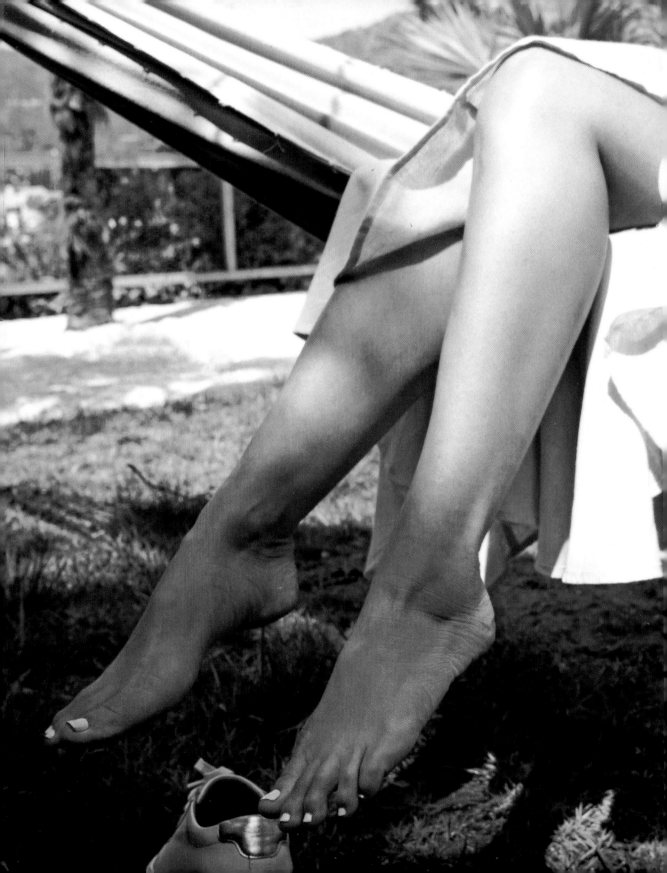

recipes for your
perfectly imperfect life

everyday ways to live and eat
for health, healing, and happiness

Kimberly Snyder, CN

HARMONY
BOOKS · NEW YORK

Published in the United States by Harmony Books, an imprint of the
Crown Publishing Group, a division of Penguin Random House LLC,
New York.
crownpublishing.com

Harmony Books is a registered trademark, and the Circle colophon is a
trademark of Penguin Random House LLC.

PHOTOGRAPH CREDITS: Ylva Erevall: cover front (*top, bottom right*);
pages 14, 24, 33, 35, 43, 62, 64, 66, 68, 72, 74, 76, 82, 89, 94, 96–97,
98, 103, 108, 111, 112–113, 114, 119, 120, 123, 131, 132–133, 137,
140, 148, 155, 158–159 (*top left, bottom right*), 160, 165, 168, 176–177
(*top, left and right*), 181, 187, 192, 195, 196, 201, 209, 210, 219, 220,
225, 228, 230–231 (*both*), 233, 234, 241, 242, 246–247, 251, 255, 263,
264. Victoria Wall Harris: cover front (*bottom left*), cover back; pages
2–3, 6, 8, 10, 22, 26, 29, 38, 41, 45, 48, 52, 56, 58, 70, 79, 87, 92, 106,
126, 134, 145, 158–159 (*top right, bottom left*), 173, 176–177 (*bottom,
left and right*), 178, 184, 188, 191, 202, 212–213, 214, 258. John
Pisani: pages 4–5. From the author's collection: pages 20, 54, 60, 81.

Library of Congress Cataloging-in-Publication Data
Names: Snyder, Kimberly, author.
Title: Recipes for your perfectly imperfect life : everyday ways to live
    and eat for health, healing, and happiness / Kimberly Snyder.
Description: New York : Harmony, 2019.
Identifiers: LCCN 2018012442 (print) | LCCN 2018021836 (ebook) |
    ISBN 9780525573722 (e-book) | ISBN 9780525573715 (hardcover)
Subjects: LCSH: Detoxification (Health) | Nutrition. | Self-care, Health.
Classification: LCC RA784.5 (ebook) | LCC RA784.5 S68 2019 (print) |
    DDC 613.2—dc23
LC record available at https://lccn.loc.gov/2018012442

ISBN 978-0-525-57371-5
Ebook ISBN 978-0-525-57372-2

Printed in the USA

Book design by Jen Wang
Cover design by Jen Wang

10 9 8 7 6 5 4 3 2

First Edition

Dedicated to my beautiful, extraordinary mother, Sally.
Yes, Mom, I picked you, and I am beyond grateful for you.
Our love is everlasting.

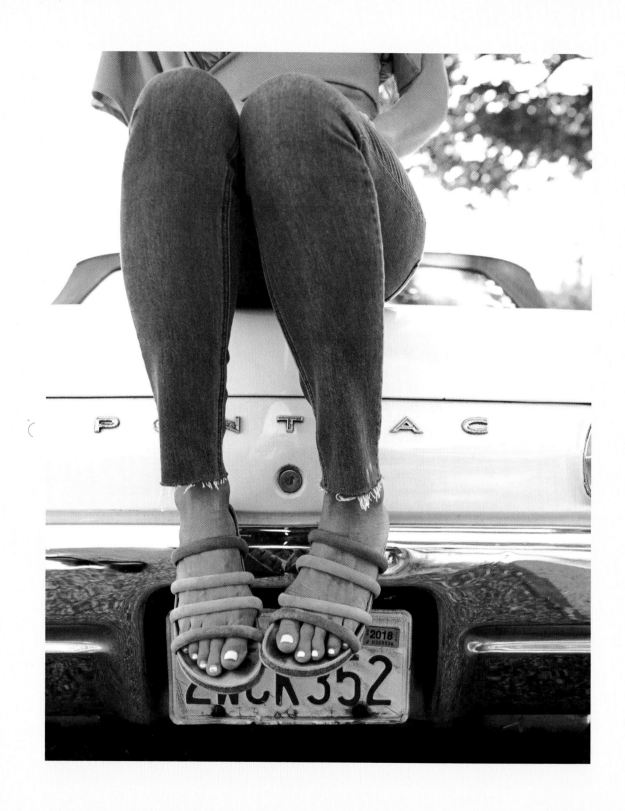

contents

part I: The Perfectly Imperfect Life — 9

part II: Recipes — 83

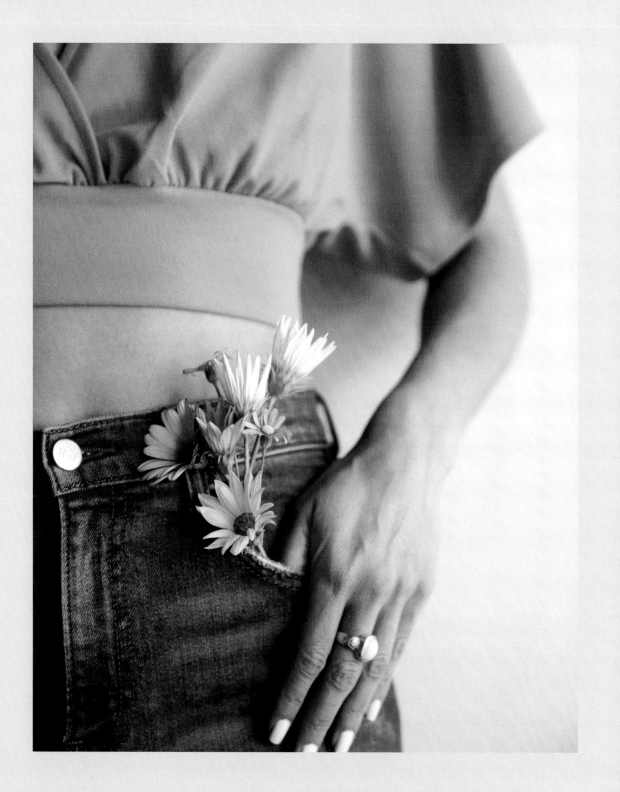

I

The
Perfectly
Imperfect
Life

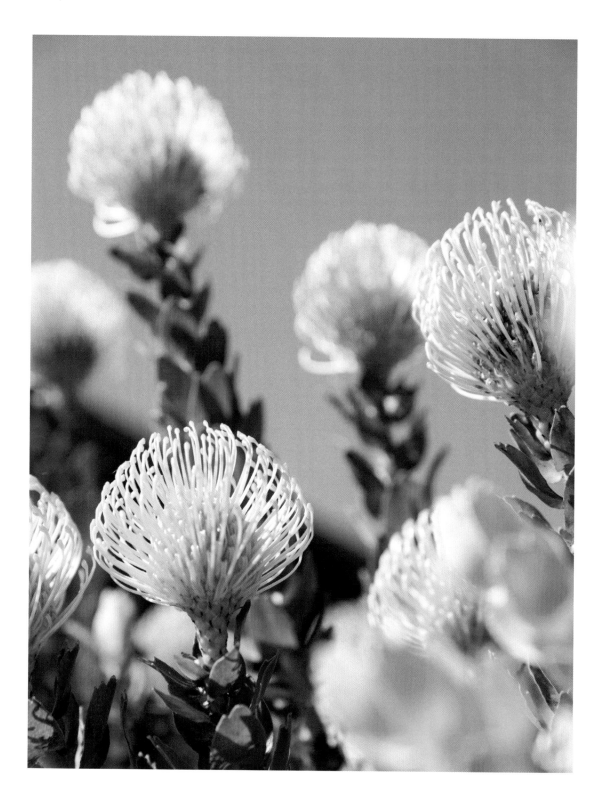

laying out the life detox plan

There's a two-thousand-year-old adage that says, "It's not what goes into a mouth that damages a person; it's what comes out of the mouth that damages a person." While I, and just about every scientist in the world, would disagree with this statement—there are plenty of carcinogens and terrible foods that do damage to our bodies—there is an element of truth to these words. No matter what we put into our bodies—organic vegetables, superfoods, the purest water—it's the thoughts we think, the words we use, and the actions we take that help define who we are and that ultimately shape our lives.

Personally, I know a lot of people who eat the best foods and have what many would call a perfect body (especially in carefully posed Instagram photos), but they aren't the nicest people. They can often be petty, mean-spirited, and downright miserable. I've also met a lot of people over the years who basically live on processed food, use toxic products, and can barely move without getting out of breath, yet they are the sweetest people with the biggest hearts. As a nutritionist, I would never want anyone to sustain themselves on junk food, but whom would you want to hang out with? I think you know what my answer would be.

I am not passing judgment, and, of course, most people aren't so polarizing. I just want to illustrate that we all have parts of us that need mending. None of us have it all. And if you pay attention to advertisement messages, clearly you'll see that marketing people know this as well. Ads may show someone who has a so-called ideal shape, a beautiful family, and flawless skin, but there is always an implied "you are missing (this one thing) . . . ," too, so companies can sell it to you and ultimately turn a profit.

I'm here to tell you that you're not missing anything. You don't even need this book, but I hope you'll read on because what I have to say is important.

Here in the West we are conditioned from an early age to think that we're imperfect on the deepest level. Sometimes that comes from advertisers, as mentioned above, sometimes from faith traditions, sometimes from the rules of society, sometimes from our own family and friends (who are also conditioned to believe they are incomplete and missing things).

But, the truth is you are perfect regardless of all the imperfections you might have. Why? Because you are alive and you are here in this very moment. The fact that you have life means you have dignity and you are part of this community we call humanity. You have the capacity to give and receive love, which is the most powerful, limitless, perfect force. The love that is inherently within you is your perfection.

It's not necessarily what we eat or how big or small our butts are, but what we *think* about ourselves and the world around us that often makes us feel connected, whole, validated, and strong. But these are just thoughts and perceptions. And guess what? Often thoughts and perceptions change in the blink of an eye. Have you ever been superhungry and moody and felt crappy about life, only to eat a fresh lunch and feel elated about something you were depressed about just an hour ago? Eating healthily and taking care of ourselves, like getting enough sleep, surely help to make us feel better in many ways. But that is not all there is to wellness.

We've learned over the past one hundred years that how and what we think influences all parts of who we are. Not only that, but simply changing the way we look at ourselves and the world around us can lead to powerful emotional, physical, and psychological transformations.

Hence, *Recipes for Your Perfectly Imperfect Life* is a guide to inner and outer transformation, which may not be instantaneous, yet it can happen relatively quickly, as we'll see in the pages ahead. This is a book that contains useful news on nutrition, life lessons, and recipes to help you embrace your perceived imperfections—whether they include being ten pounds over your desired weight, having a too-large nose or rough skin, being easily annoyed or not assertive enough, not being in the "right" place in your career or family life, or simply not feeling good enough. Ultimately, I want you to experience the perfection already present in you and in your life. This book will teach you how to stay anchored to a permanent inner source of power, allowing you to clear "life blocks" so you can experience your most beautiful life.

Part I includes a number of Life Detox Recipes, which are practical tips about life and food drawn from my own personal stories and those of people I have worked with over the years (with names changed for privacy, of course). These are offered to detox your life on a deeper level, helping you break through emotional and mental blocks that have an effect not only on your physical health and beauty but also on your ability to be truly happy. I share some of my most vulnerable parts with you on my bumpy path to self-acceptance, including through the stories of my son's not-as-planned birth story, showing emotion in public, and rehabbing the perfectionist addict in me. This is all in an effort to show you that life can sometimes be a mess (that is, I can be a mess!). And that's okay, because it's in that mess that we discover who we are.

Part II includes more than one hundred delicious recipes that are nutrient-dense, energizing, cleansing, and nourishing on many levels. All these recipes are plant-based, gluten-free, and properly food combined, a concept based in making digestion easier in order to free up more energy (see page 84 for more info). No matter your current diet, working these recipes into your life is an easy, surefire way to raise your vitality, health, and happiness. Last, if you want to learn more about the studies, articles, and books I mention in *Recipes for Your Perfectly Imperfect Life,* go to mysolluna.com for details.

I'm so excited to be on this journey with you. Detoxing self-doubt and confusion clears the way for you to enjoy your amazing, delicious, perfectly imperfect life more than you ever realized possible.

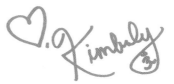

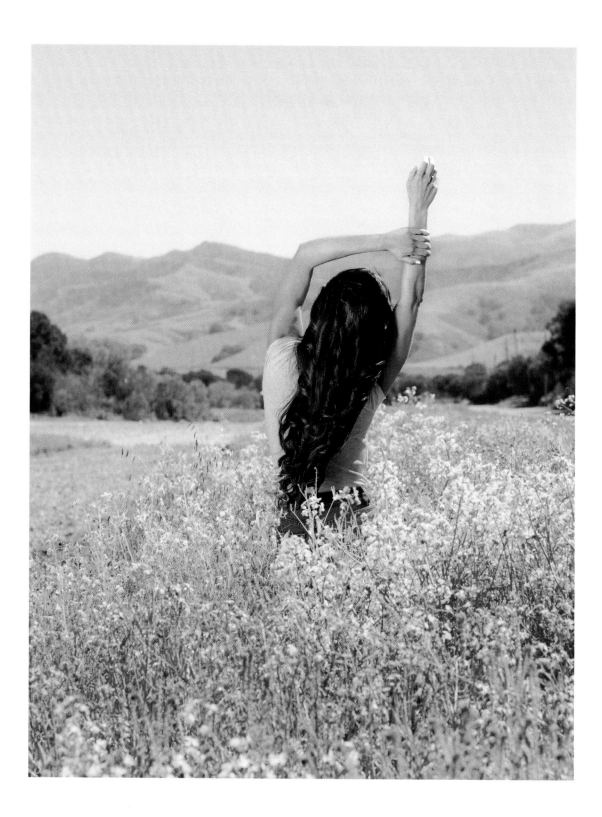

If you want to become whole: Unless you accept yourself,
you can't let go of yourself.
—Stephen Mitchell's notes on Lao-tzu's *Tao Te Ching*, chapter 21

CHAPTER 1

clearing the blocks that hold us back

An "And" Life

We live in a world overrun by the word *or*. Traditionally, we've been taught to classify things as one or the other. Good *or* bad. Healthy *or* not. Fat *or* skinny. Beautiful *or* average. This small word might not seem like a big deal, but it dictates the way we think, experience, and ultimately embrace or reject the world around us. But we don't have to buy into an "either/or" existence. Instead, we can shift to the all-encompassing word *and*.

Our life journeys may go pretty well sometimes, like the days when we hit all the green lights and get a promotion at work and top it off with a superfun night out with friends. And sometimes not so much. Big challenges often pop up, we fall off track, and some days nothing seems to go our way. Life is certainly not black or white. We drink Glowing Green Smoothies (aka GGS; page 99) and sometimes eat too many cupcakes when we get stressed at work. We can be both happy and sad, depending on the moment. We can be calm and sometimes reactive. We can be healthy and also in need of healing.

When we embrace an "and" life, we don't have to feel bad when we screw up, nor do we have to judge ourselves or others because what often seems like contradiction is all part of our journey to wholeness. Eating that cupcake doesn't invalidate our pursuit of health— we can choose to follow rhythms of eating clean *and* we can enjoy a dessert.

The "either/or" mentality pushes us to judge everything, to slot things into categories. Being overly judgmental does not feel good to any of us. When we're constantly judging, we feel tense and restless instead of calm and peaceful. This doesn't mean we shouldn't have opinions, nor does it mean we shouldn't try to make good decisions or stand for a cause. It just means we do our best and reserve our opinions. We can be humble, knowing that we don't know the whole picture of what's "right," for us or anyone else. Lao-tzu's *Tao Te Ching* teaches us "Do your work, then step back." Think about some events in life you have experienced that seemed like a disaster at the time, which then turned out to be good for you. Maybe a relationship spontaneously combusted. You felt terrible. You thought your world was over. Your mind just kept going

in circles, and you thought life would never be the same.

Then after a few months and a lot of tumbling over your own emotions (and crying into your pillow), you meet someone who turns out to be, for lack of a better phrase, your soul mate. You never would have met that person if you were still in your previous relationship. Or maybe you experienced the flip side. Say you started working at your dream job and you felt like all the stars aligned, and then after a few weeks, it turns out that your dream job is really a nightmare. What you thought was the best thing in the world turned out to be not so great after all.

Like many things, our judgments can sometimes set up impossible standards that prevent us from seeing clearly or acting in ways that are beneficial to us. Think how much better it feels to observe what's in front of you without making a negative passing comment, without casting a verdict. Some of you may be balking now. You might think passing judgment doesn't really affect your life in a negative way, or maybe you even get a rise out of it. But for a moment, contrast how it feels on a rainy day when you just observe the clouds and rain falling outside your window with how it feels when you look on the same scene but you're angry or depressed because you had hoped for a sunny day.

Yoga master Paramahansa Yogananda teaches us that constantly comparing what you like against what you don't like is a major cause of suffering. Again, I don't mean that you shouldn't get excited or have great expectations about things in your life. I'm not saying you should be some kind of robot, but life can feel so much more relaxed and happy when we embrace a world that can be many things at the same time, including imperfect and perfect.

A New Way of Looking at Perfection

All of us, no matter who we are, from celebrities to working moms and dads, are undeniably flawed. We make mistakes, say the wrong thing, we're moody, sometimes we act inappropriately or have emotional meltdowns; we might drink too much or obsess over what we eat all day instead of focusing on a work project; we might show a happy face in front of the people we work with and then criticize them to our friend over dinner; or flip someone off on the highway and let loose a diatribe of obscenities that would make our granny have a heart attack.

But just as we are undeniably flawed, we are also undeniably perfect.

Not perfect in the way the word *perfect* is popularly used. As in *Her hair is so perfect. She has such a perfect life. Everyone in spin class has such a perfect body. He has the perfect job.* These are all self-imposed standards for defining perfection that change with the times. Like trends, they are ephemeral and seasonal, here today and gone tomorrow. Just a few years ago, perfection for a woman was defined as someone who was superskinny. For at least ten years, almost all jean companies promoted the skinny jean, a pair of pants that fit only a small demographic of the population. Today, media trends seem to have changed all that. Now, for some, a "perfect" body is curvy with a big, rounded butt that would never fit into a pair of classic skinny jeans (unless they are superstretchy in the bottom!). So-called physical perfection in this sense is really just judgment in the eye of the beholder or selfie/belfie taker. Why hold ourselves to a standard that is simultaneously fleeting, impossible, and arbitrary?

Yet no matter what we look like or how screwed up our lives might be financially, professionally, psycho- logically, or even spiritually, it doesn't take away from the fact that we are alive in the here and now. Just the fact that you have life, that you are a breathing, feeling, thinking creature who laughs and cries and eats and moves in some way means you are perfect. There is an essence, a true and good essence, that is the center of who we are. This ability to empathize, connect, and love others means there is perfect love inside you. This can be hard to accept because of all the conditioning humans have gone through during millions of years of social evolution, but it's a truth that I am living by now in my own life.

I mean, think about this: What makes you imperfect? Maybe you think your eyes are too close together. Who ever said eyes need to be a certain distance apart? Who made that decision? Maybe you were born with a learning disability and other people looked at you judgmentally while you were growing up. Who said that learning in a different way makes you imperfect? Who? Seriously, I want names. Maybe your parents called you plain or said you weren't good enough while you were growing up? No offense, but who are these people and who made them experts on what's beautiful or not? Why listen to that BS?

So maybe you don't wake up at 6 a.m. to work out every day, maybe you don't finish your to-do list every day, maybe you only get through one day of the 30 Day Roadmap (our Solluna healthy-eating video course), maybe you make mistakes at work, maybe you don't reach every deadline. Take all of this in stride. I don't care about the size of your bank account or social media following, or what you look like or what your job title is. I don't care if you're overweight or have ripped abs; none

the amazing wisdom of our bodies

Some approaches to nutrition prescribe dozens and dozens of supplements to make up for all that is "missing." And while the right nutrients are, of course, key, we achieve true vitality and wellness by supporting our bodies in doing what they naturally know to do. We need to remove obstructions like toxins, chemicals, and pesticides that keep our bodies from working their best. There is a big difference between hyperfocusing on what's missing versus focusing on supporting the natural intelligence of our bodies.

One of the most effective ways for us to support our bodies is to optimize our digestion with the right kinds of probiotics, digestive enzymes, and oxygen cleanse aids. These help us absorb nutrients more efficiently, which, in turn, elevates our energy, health, and moods. Ongoing detoxification protocols, which include eating a fiber-rich, totally or largely plant-based diet, are also important, yet they are just as much about cleansing out what weighs us down as the nutrients they supply.

of it makes you better or worse than anyone else. What matters is that you have a heart, not just the organ that beats in your body but an essence that is connected to something greater than us. Sure we can always improve our lives. I mean, that's what I've dedicated my life's work toward: helping others to feel better physically and emotionally. Yet regardless of our so-called flaws,

we are already whole, with a vast storehouse of potential inside us to expand that wholeness in order to become truly happy and healthy and to help the world be a better place.

Now let's turn our attention to our "imperfections." What am I talking about when I use this word? Our imperfections are our quirks, survival techniques, coping mechanisms—all the ways that we are working things out on our journey. These can include impatience, stormy behaviors, a tendency to be envious, the inability to express our needs clearly or to let go of pain or resentment, or bursting into tears at any kind of confrontation. We're all in process. We make mistakes, hopefully learn from them, and make new mistakes. So what? Keep moving forward!

When we feel bad about our imperfections, guilt, shame, anger, anxiety, and poor body image come into play. When we think that we have to be something other than what we are, we disconnect from ourselves and from others, and from everyday aspects of life, including our food and diets.

Don't get me wrong. I don't think we should be needy, irritating, or emotional basket cases who spill our negative feelings all over other people. We need to carry ourselves with strength and dignity. Food is an easy target to offload our bad feelings about ourselves and our bodies, and it can all too easily become enemies and weapons that punish and control us. Yet when we feel content with our perfect imperfection, we feel motivated to make healthy life choices, and food and diet become ways of self-care and self-nourishment.

So, here's a little homework. It will take just a minute or two. Think of things that stress you out. Maybe you had a child a couple of years ago and can't get rid of that mom belly. Or maybe you're so worried about money

life recipes

One of the most powerful things we can do is to embrace the idea that we are *both* perfect and imperfect. We are inherently alive with a body that ages and transforms over time. But we also carry within us an essence, a part of us that is perfect and unchangeable. All of us have imperfections. We might screw things up from time to time, but we are all on a journey to discover the love and true essence at the core of who we are. Although we've been taught that things have to be one or the other, actually these two states coexist within each of us.

Choosing to live an "and" life means holding our judgment in check. This is for us and for others. An "and" approach to life is inclusive and feels open and free. Thinking that things have to be one way or another is polarizing and stressful. Who needs that? We can choose to let all that kind of thinking go, and feel happier.

life detox recipes

We can all live with our challenges and imperfections, yet still lead a life that is centered, balanced, and connected to ourselves and others.

When we start to feel a little off-balance, a great self-care practice is to eat a cleansing and nurturing soup, which is full of easily digested nutrients, as well as fiber and liquid to help you feel satisfied and present within your body without feeling heavy.

Here are two particularly great options:

» GINGER CABBAGE CLEANSE SOUP (page 163). This soup contains ginger, a warming spice to enact digestive and energetic change. Cabbage has natural detoxifying properties and nourishes your gut while reducing inflammation.

» CURRIED RADIANCE CARROT SOUP (page 164). This soup is packed with beta-carotene-rich carrots grown deep down in the earth, the food equivalent of "earthing," or balancing our energy through connecting with nature's energy, as well as spices and herbs that improve circulation and integration of nutrients.

you lie awake until 2 a.m. every night. Where can you embrace "and" over "or"? For example, can't you still be and feel beautiful *and* carry a few extra pounds around with you? Can you be concerned about your finances *and* still be funny and outgoing? Try to look at opposing parts of your life and personality, and instead of saying something has to be "either/or," see if you can use an "and" mentality. Loosen the grip on labeling issues as one thing or another, and see how much more peaceful your life becomes.

My Journey to Healing

Ever look at someone who is successful professionally or personally or socially, or whatever, and secretly ask how she seems to have it all together? We compare their lives to ours, at least as their lives appear to us in social media and on paper, and lament how our life is unglamorous, messed up, and boring in comparison.

I've had my own level of success. I've been more than fortunate. Throughout the years some people have said to me how amazing it is that I have it all figured out. I always chuckle when I hear this. While anyone can read about my public life online, it doesn't reflect the whole story at all. For all the legitimate smiles and excitement, my life is like any other life. I doubt things, feel insecure, struggle to love myself, and still occasionally feel body shame.

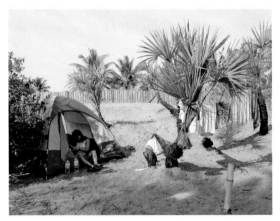

Camping in Mozambique during my around-the-world journey.

As I've shared in my first book, *The Beauty Detox Solution*, and on my website, for a few years I was on an intense path of learning as I journeyed around the world. The wandering was reflective of what was going on in my mind, which was deeply searching and seeking and questioning pretty much everything I had ever believed—from what I knew about food (at the time I was a hard-core calorie and protein-gram counter) to spirituality (I was raised Catholic and had never tried meditation or yoga or been exposed to Eastern philosophy at that point) to what success in life really meant. You could say I was on a kind of vision quest, though I had not preplanned for that to happen.

I ended up traveling far and wide, working in Australia, then backpacking the world for about three years. I camped across Africa for months, living in a tent and cooking with a camping stove, traveling in a beat-up car, zigzagged across China on third-class trains, lived in shack-like bungalows in Southeast Asia without electricity or running water, practiced yoga in ashrams across the Himalayas and along the Ganges, meditated at Buddhist temples, slept on the floors of random families' *gers* (nomadic tents) when I explored the Gobi Desert in Mongolia, and trekked around ruins, floating islands, and rain forests in South America. I summited Mount Kilimanjaro, climbed the Huangshan mountain in China, and hiked the Annapurna trek in Nepal.

I immersed myself in local cultures, often using my hands, smiles, and music for communication, and I committed myself to discovering wellness, dietary, and beauty practices everywhere I was. Yet I still had no idea (and I mean *zero* idea) how the rest of my life was going to turn out and how I was going to translate all the amazing knowledge I was absorbing into a career.

I moved to New York City after my world travels, totally broke yet bursting with passion. I started my blog and continued to learn about nutrition. There was a transition period when I had to be superscrappy and take many kinds of jobs to pay for my tiny rent-stabilized apartment. This was all before I studied to become a nutritionist, built up a client list, landed my first book deal, and created a whole lifestyle philosophy. During this period, there was tremendous self-doubt and insomnia. I questioned whether I had messed up my life by not getting a "real" job right when I graduated, like everyone else I knew from college.

Besides my nutrition work, I taught group and private yoga classes part of the time, and even in the dead of winter, I would walk thirty or forty minutes to get to the next client, as there were months when I couldn't pay for an unlimited subway ticket. I also worked at a raw food café in the East Village and had a brief stint in real estate and an even shorter one in multilevel marketing with my mom, which involved Japanese water and air filters. Totally random, I know! I once took an office job at a large beauty company. I despised the company culture—what the whole company stood for—and I was bored with my daily tasks. I lasted only three months.

I was on a panel recently and was asked how I pulled through hard times when beginning my career. My answer is that even when I was starting out, a freshly landed backpacker hustling to survive in fast, unrelenting New York City, I kept helping others as the central focus of my work. I started my blog to share with others how to feel their best. Whenever I wrote an article or gave a talk or taught a class, I stayed connected to giving to each and every reader or listener. And looking back, when I faltered from that and started overworrying about the business part, everything suffered.

So no, I don't have "it" figured out, but I do genuinely believe that keeping the focus on service and love has helped me actualize my dreams. It translated into cocreating the vision of my life, which includes writing books, building an incredible wellness community, and founding and running Solluna, a business where I get to develop products and content I love and am honored to offer to our community and world. And I get to work from home so I can take care of my young son.

On the deepest level, beyond what I was *doing* in the world, my own inner healing journey has been ongoing. It started with my around-the-world journey. It has accelerated in the past few years as I've confronted life at its very core, experiencing the birth of my first child and the passing of my mother.

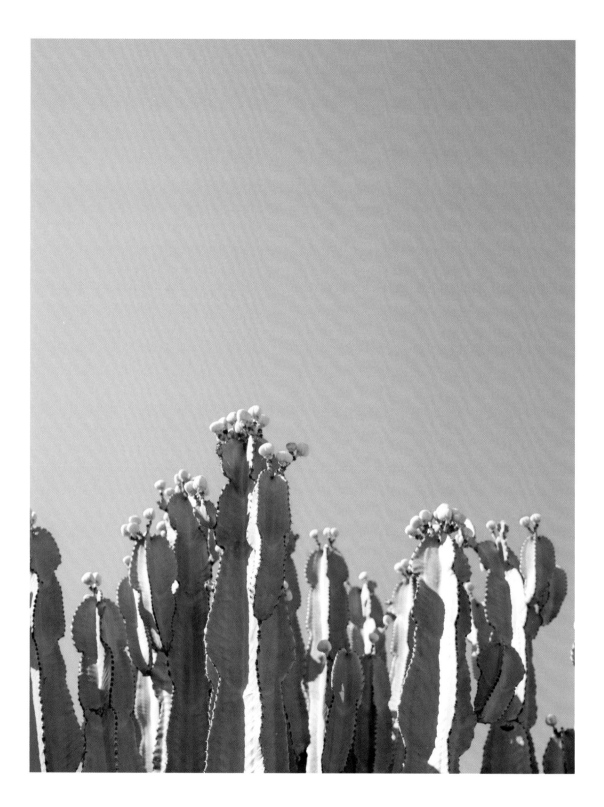

Your Incredible Journey

You, too, are on a one-of-a-kind journey, unlike anyone else's. There is real power in acknowledging the uniqueness that *is* you, and the stamp of your life. You are your most beautiful when you apologetically own your life and get comfortable with the fact that no one else can walk your path. It is yours, and no one else can be you. Comparing or trying to look or be like someone else only waters down your power and unique beauty.

We've been taught to hide parts of ourselves: to project a "perfect" image by looking a certain way and appearing to have it all figured out.

life detox recipe
Since including the good of others in your goals and aspirations will help actualize your own dreams into reality, try making big, nourishing one-pot or baked meals to share. It feels great and helps to boost things energetically in a positive direction for you.

Here are two excellent recipes to share from one big pot or container:

» ONE-POT LOVE CHILI (page 183). Full of protein, minerals, fiber, and antioxidants, this is an easy meal to put together, along with your love, and dish it up for a crowd.

» JAMAICAN SOUL FOOD SHEPHERD'S PIE (page 189). This is a nourishing recipe full of nutrient-dense veggies and digestion-stimulating herbs and spices, including anise and cumin, and calming, blood-sugar-balancing coriander.

When we spend all this energy concealing some parts and dressing up other parts of our lives, it's exhausting. And we then overly stress about our imperfections, because we are putting so much focus on the surface parts of our lives. Yet if we shift to staying more connected to the perfection inside of us, to the love that connects us to everything else, our appearances don't seem direly serious.

It's not that we don't care about how we look or what we do—because for sure we do. It's just that we can be so much more comfortable and joyful within ourselves day to day. And that's what really counts: if we define success in life by how truly happy we are. Sure, we can display a "perfect" job, house, marriage, body, and so on on the outside, yet if we are miserable deep down, does any of that really matter? Others can sense this shift in us, this increasing sense of ease, and it starts a chain reaction for others to be more accepting of themselves, too. We can help make the world become brighter and lighter, starting with ourselves.

It's a simple yet big concept to really embody. Keep reading, because the ideas and practices we discuss in our journey together throughout this book are going to help you integrate the truth of how amazing and good enough you truly are, once and for all.

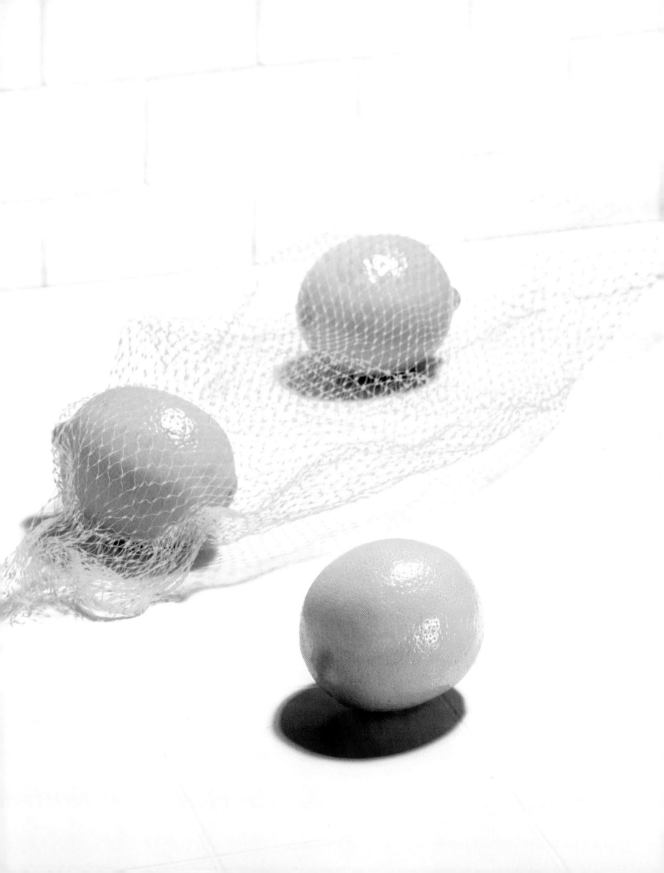

Morning Practice

DRINK HOT WATER WITH LEMON: This simple, powerful practice helps to cleanse and detoxify your system. Lemons supply vitamin C, as well as enzymes that help regenerate your liver tissue.

MEDITATION OR STILLNESS PRACTICE: This can take many forms, from simply listening to your breath, praying, setting intentions, practicing meditative techniques to following a *sadhana*, or a daily spiritual practice. Whatever form you like, commit to this "you time" in the morning, which connects you to your body and self, and can help with everything from warding off food cravings to being more in tune with your true hunger and nutritional needs. It also helps you feel more centered throughout the ups and downs of the day, and supports your overall vitality by supporting a healthy adrenal and nervous system.

Stillness also helps us connect back with the whole, and the Oneness of which we are a part.

SOIL-BASED ORGANISM (SBO) PROBIOTICS: A healthy gut is a huge key to feeling balanced and achieving well-being. Yet probiotics are not all created equal! Many formulas are denatured by the time you even take them, offer only a small percentage of the bacterium we need for balance, or take the "kitchen sink" approach, meaning just a bit of this and that to sound good for marketing. SBOs mimic the perfect bacterial mix found in the healthy soil that our ancestors used to consume on unwashed vegetables and fruit. SBOs are a natural, powerful way to get probiotics, as they are hearty enough to survive stomach acid and implant in our guts.

I'm so unbelievably passionate about probiotics that I created my own proprietary SBO formula with the best ratios of clinically researched strains to support a healthy gut flora. This formula is especially powerful in fostering increased energy, vitality, focus, and immunity; improving digestion; detoxifying environmental toxins; and creating better hair, skin, and a higher quality of life all around. For more information, please visit my website.

THE GLOWING GREEN SMOOTHIE (AKA GGS): This is my signature elixir, which supplies you with vital antioxidants, vitamins, minerals, cleaning fiber, and countless other micronutrients. It gives you an incredible amount of sustained energy, detoxifies toxins from your system, and supports glowing skin. I encourage you to mix and match your greens and fruit, but stick with the basic ratio of around 70 percent greens and 30 percent fruit and vitamin C and detox-boosting lemon juice (yes, more lemon!) in the classic GGS recipe (page 99).

life detox recipe

One of the most powerful ways to set yourself up for a great day is to anchor yourself to a defined morning practice. Often, we start the day already frazzled and disconnected from ourselves. We reach for our phone first thing, and our minds are already on work and the tasks ahead while we scarf down a protein bar or an egg-white omelet, barely chewing and feeling mounting anxiety that we are already behind.

In contrast, a consistent morning rhythm gets you into a good flow. You will start off the beginning of each day feeling strong, clear of physical and emotional blocks, energized, poised, and focused.

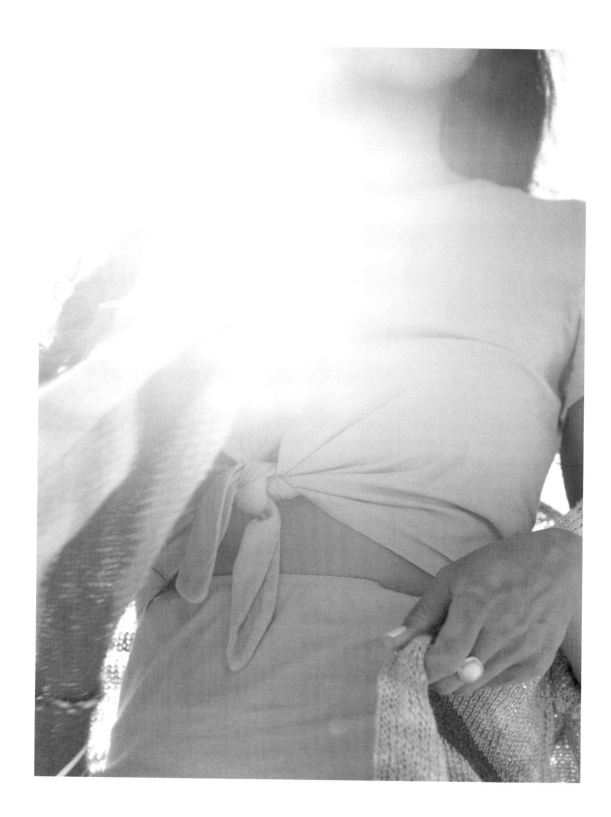

CHAPTER 2

flowing (rather than drowning)

Imposter in Rome

Do you remember the last time you got caught showing a side of yourself that you were not proud of? As much as we try to carefully filter what we show our family and friends, and colleagues at work, and on social media, we can't filter all of life. Many of us have the tendency to feel ashamed when we don't look the way we'd like to in certain moments. Yet even in those sticky situations, we all have opportunities to choose to be authentic and vulnerable and real.

I'd like to share a personal story about this. I love bumping into my readers and Solluna community members all around the world and sharing hugs. But when I was in Rome a few years ago, I ran into a reader during a painfully awkward moment.

I was in Europe working with clients and decided to take a weekend trip to the Eternal City with my significant other. We got in some silly fight walking between the Colosseum and the Pantheon. The issue was small and petty, but I was stubbornly holding on to the annoyance and our little spat dragged on.

We were right in the middle of the argument, and I had just said something pretty nasty. My face was scrunched into a tight ball. My partner walked away from me. Right then, a sweet brown-haired woman wearing a blue cardigan with a little seven- or eight-year-old girl in tow came up to me and said, "Oh, you're Kimberly Snyder! I have your books on my nightstand!"

My first instinct was sheer panic. Had she heard me arguing? Would she think I was actually an awful person in real life? I couldn't let that happen! I was too terrified of looking bad. In that state of panic, I blurted out, "No, you must have mistaken me for someone else." The woman cocked her head in a puzzled way, and I darted away.

I let a full minute go by, scurrying in the other direction. Then it sank in what I had done. I had lied! *I pretended I wasn't me!* All because I was ashamed I would possibly be seen as a mean person who gets into fights. A side of me that I didn't want to let my readers—or anyone except for those closest to me—ever see.

It hit me: I can't let this happen! I can't be some fake. I spun around and ran to catch up with the woman. Now she was walking down the promenade with both her daughter and her husband. I took a deep breath. This was going to be painful.

Practice authenticity across your life. Use good judgment and don't lie. This includes not only your relationships with friends, family, and colleagues, but also your relationship with food. There may be foods that you love that might not always be the healthiest for you. If you really love sandwiches, for instance, it might feel more authentic to find a bridge by eating them sometimes versus eating *only* salads. If you make a drastic switch to the latter and try to use sheer willpower and go against your true feelings all the time, it might erupt into falling off the wagon altogether.

The key is finding healthy alternatives for what you love that are easily digested and cleansing, yet still delicious and satisfying. Yes, it is possible to have both! Try it for yourself and become a believer in healthier upgrades that still keep you feeling excited about your food. It takes many of us a long time to transition off certain foods (it took me two whole years to give up cheese), and that's okay.

Here are some great food alternatives for old classics:

》 The delicious LOVE THYME VEGGIE BURGER (page 203) offers a nutrient-dense patty full of protein and minerals such as iron. It is an excellent replacement for beef hamburgers, which are full of various toxins, including antibiotics, steroids, mycotoxins, heavy metals, dioxins, and other forms of industrial pollutants (some of these are even present in organic meat). Try making larger batches and freezing extras to eat when you are in a time bind.

》 If you love Mexican food (and who doesn't, really?!), check out the EASY SWEET POTATO AND PINTO BEAN ENCHILADAS (page 198), which are salsa-y and have both creamy and "meaty" textures, yet without any dairy or processed ground meat or chicken.

》 The ALL VEGGIE CLEAN LASAGNA (page 185) is stuffed with so many delicious ingredients and fillings. It contains none of the greasy dairy, meat, or gluten . . . or even any kind of noodles for that matter!

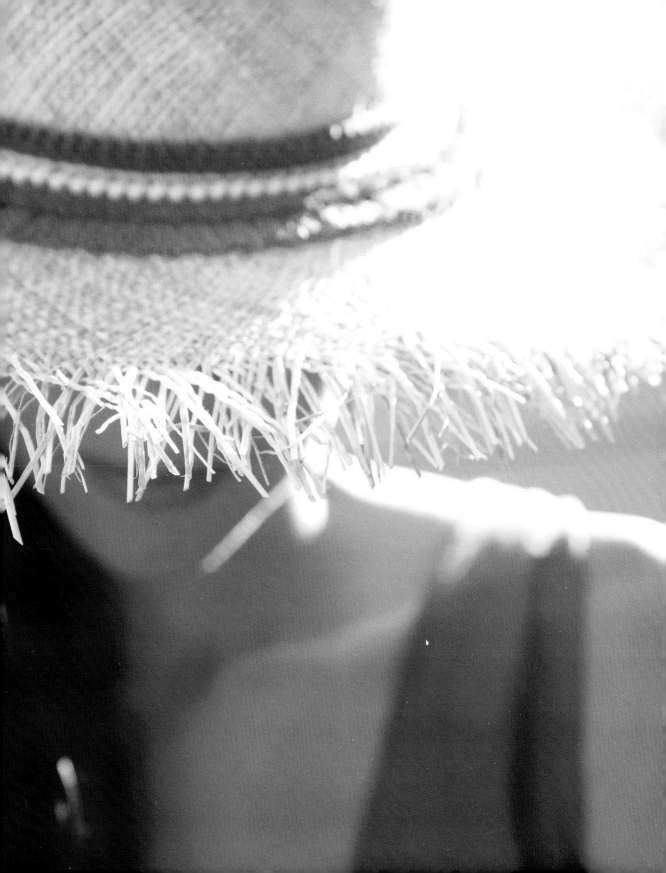

"Oh, hi there! I'm so sorry, I actually am Kimberly!"

I explained I had been utterly embarrassed because I had been bickering with my partner. She and her husband laughed, joking that they "might know a thing or two about that!" She accepted my apology and said how relieved she was that I fessed up, because she *knew* it was me.

I talked to them for about ten minutes, and we had a great connection. As I walked away, I shook my head . . . so much weirdness and drama, all of which *I* created. The lesson I learned from this superawkward encounter is that it's okay to be a real person instead of pretending that all of life is perfect.

Consider the moments in your life that you're less than proud of. It could just as easily have been you having it out with your sister or mom, let's say, at the grocery store, when an old friend from college or a colleague from your last job approached you at that exact moment. Or maybe you were squabbling with the manager at Target about some returns, and things started to get heated when the new guy you just started seeing sidled up. Or you snap at your partner in front of the neighbors. While such situations are not ones we strive for, we also don't want to internalize guilt so much that we start feeling bad about ourselves. We're complex, whole beings, and we're going to have good days and bad days. Messy moments are part of the imperfect journey of growth in life. Acknowledge the mess, learn, and move on.

life detox recipe

Being phony and hiding and pretending is much worse than being real, even when we think we look bad. Next time you have the urge to give a fake smile to your friend when you feel awful, or to deny that you overreacted to a pretty innocuous comment that your boyfriend made, lean in to the feeling, staying curious as to why something might have bothered you so much. It's brave—and ultimately freeing—to confront the parts of ourselves we wouldn't normally broadcast at dinner parties or on social media. Find some private space if need be, and cry if you feel like it. Finding healthy ways to process feelings instead of repressing them is part of being authentic.

The Feelings-Inflammation Link

Inflammation is a vital part of our body's immune response and a way to heal itself. We've all experienced acute inflammation, marked by short-term redness, swelling, warmth, or pain that arises with a cut or a scrape, a twisted ankle, or the flu.

Yet there is another type of inflammation, which is the modern epidemic of chronic, low-grade inflammation. This type destroys the balance in our bodies and lowers our vitality, making us more susceptible to diseases that range from autoimmune conditions to heart disease, elevated white blood cell count, diabetes, and more. Low-grade inflammation can also show up as acne, wrinkles, candidiasis, acid reflux, and chronic pain.

So what causes this awful chronic inflammation? First of all, diet plays a huge role. Excess sugar and refined sugar is a big offender. Yet so is a diet high in animal protein. The journal *Nutrition* reports that those who ate protein from meat had higher levels of inflammation compared to participants who consumed mostly fish or plant-based sources of protein. And a 2015 study in the journal *Nutrients* found a positive effect on glucose levels when people switched from animal to plant protein. We don't want to overdo protein in general; research has shown excess protein creates an elevated response to insulin similar to that of excess carbs, for roughly the same period of time, which may come as a surprise to many of us.

It's also important to balance fat, and to eat healthy types over fried or rancid forms, as research has shown that a high-fat meal—but not a high-carbohydrate meal—is associated with subsequent increases in plasma IL-6, an inflammation marker. Other causes of chronic, low-grade inflammation include food allergies, food sensitivities, dysbiosis (imbalance in gut flora), environmental toxicity (including from heavy metals), and a lack of sleep.

The Beauty Detox/Solluna philosophy, outlined in my prior Beauty Detox books and throughout the Solluna website and offerings, is naturally anti-inflammatory in its dietary approach, as it is balanced in its levels of protein, fat, and carbohydrates, and is based in nutrient-dense, fibrous plant foods and devoid of gluten, dairy, saturated-fat-containing meat, junk foods, processed

life detox recipe

Eating to support digestion and gut balance is critical for helping to avoid physical and emotional inflammation in your body. Here are some great recipes to support this:

» CUMIN ROASTED BRUSSELS SPROUTS WITH QUINOA (page 194). This dish is full of plant-based protein, which digests cleanly and doesn't add to toxicity buildup. We can easily obtain our entire protein needs from an all or largely plant-based diet without overdoing protein. *Too much* protein makes us overly acidic and is associated with cancer and many health problems. This is the real issue—not too little protein!

» ENERGIZING PISTACHIO HEMPSEED CUCUMBER SALAD WITH ORANGE ZEST (page 115). This salad supplies us with omega-3 fats via delicious, earthy-tasting hempseeds, which help reduce inflammation by balancing our essential fatty acid (EFA) ratio.

» THE GLOWING GREEN SMOOTHIE (aka GGS; page 99). Dehydration contributes to inflammation, so stay hydrated with the vitamin- and nutrient-dense GGS, as well as drinking plenty of room temperature water and coconut water. Avoid sodas and too much caffeine.

and heated vegetable oils, and refined sugars. It includes dark leafy greens and chia, hemp-, and flaxseeds, which are all important sources of anti-inflammatory omega-3 fatty acids.

Yet beyond how we eat and sleep, a growing body of research is now proving how much our *emotions* impact inflammation and how, in turn, the more inflamed our bodies are, the worse we feel. A 2015 study found that people with depression had 30 percent more brain inflammation than those who were not depressed. Our physical and emotional-mental states of being are really one whole that affects every part of us, though we often treat them as separate.

Negative feelings can and *do* create pain and disease and accelerate aging. A paper titled "Stress, Negative Emotions, and Inflammation" overviews how stress, depression, anger, hostility, and negative emotions "appear to promote the production of inflammatory mediators, providing a physiological mechanism by which negative psychological states may impact health." A study in *JAMA Psychiatry* found that those who exhibited explosive anger had higher levels of inflammatory markers, such as C-reactive proteins (CRP). Road rage and heated family battles can really come back to bite us.

Research demonstrates that our hearts, the sensitive organ that not only physically pumps blood but is the area in our bodies where we deeply sense love and emotions, is as affected by our feelings as by what is on our plate. A study of Mexican-American women found a correlation between anger and hostility with inflammation and heart disease, and similar research backs up anger expression as a predictor of cardiovascular disease. In contrast, a 2017 study from the journal *Emotion* entitled "Emodiversity and Biomarkers of Inflammation" found that positive emotions are associated with lower circulat-

ing levels of inflammation. The takeaway? Taking care of our emotions is as critical to our health and well-being and warding off inflammation as eating properly!

So how do we take care of our emotions? First of all, let them be felt and processed in real time instead of pushing them down. Repression accumulates a brewing, energy-zapping storehouse of negativity, albeit beneath the surface, and can inflame us in a parallel way to chemical pesticides. This mass of emotional toxins contributes to continual stress and anxiety-induced meltdowns.

Have you ever seen a kid fall on the playground, followed by the mom running over saying, "You're okay! You're okay!" She's obviously coming from the loving space of trying to quell her child's fears (and her own). But really, how does she know the kid is okay? She's telling her child how she feels, instead of letting the child express and feel that pain.

I used to act the same way. When I started going to infant classes with Lil' Bub (my nickname for my son), I was guided by the instructor to simply narrate what happened, as in "You tripped over Bailey's foot" or "You bumped your head on that toy you didn't see" instead of trying to soothe him with that very same "You're okay!" It didn't seem natural at first, but once I retrained myself not to *tell* him his feelings, it started to really resonate. Pushing down or glossing over feelings is an instinct many of us have unknowingly inherited, and we perpetuate it in our own children.

As adults, when we're feeling upset and someone says, "You're fine," we might want to tell them to buzz off (to say it politely), because we are *not* okay at that moment. We don't want our problems to be glossed over or fixed. We are not looking for solutions right then. We are simply looking to express our emotions. As humans, it's healthy for us to experience the range of feelings that we

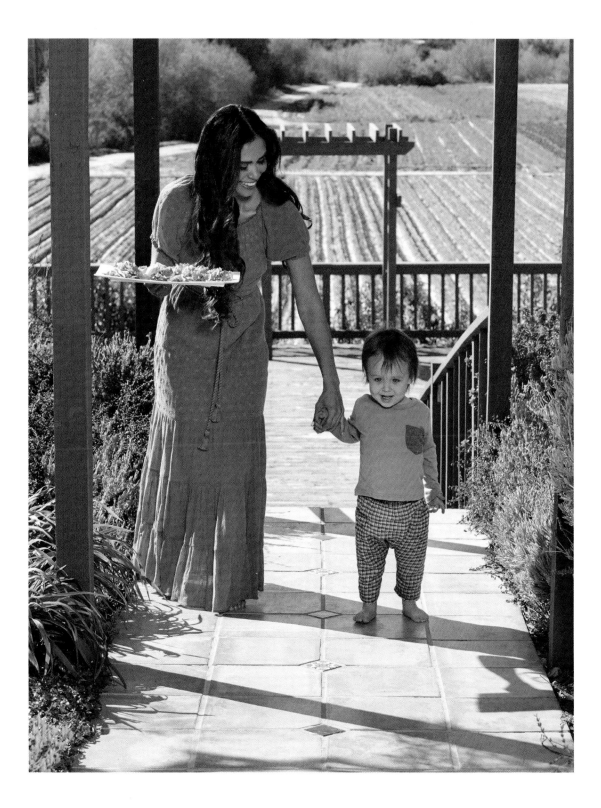

do. Often we just need some time to process them until the big feelings subside, and then in our own time, lift our faces out of the hands we've been sobbing into, and get up and carry on.

life detox recipe

It's important to experience your feelings. Meditation is a great ongoing tool for being more centered long-term. Yet life is messy and imperfect, and when stuff comes up during the day that pisses us off or upsets us, practice the Stumbling Block Detox (at right) and also the Letting Go technique (page 42) in real time, which puts your focus squarely on your emotions as they come up, to prevent emotional blocks and physical inflammation. Keep reading!

So the next time some big feelings come up, try not to push them down, or put on a fake happy face, or project the negativity outward by venting your frustration toward a poor cashier at the gas station or at your little brother. Simply try to be okay with whatever you're feeling, knowing that whatever you are experiencing is more often than not temporary. If we don't acknowledge our feelings now, emotional inflammation, anger, and sadness will create toxic blocks inside of us.

As you can tell, detoxing and processing negative emotions plays a crucial role in our well-being, alongside healthy diet and lifestyle measures. We may have been taught to shy away from pain and sadness. Yet now we can mature and stop pretending that it's all okay when it's not, and feel what is there, even if it sucks. There is a real heaviness in carrying around negative emotions, and when you consciously unpack that load, you will free up a tidal wave of energy that can be rechanneled toward elevating your health and vitality.

life detox recipe

Start to break the pattern of limiting beliefs that screw with your life with the Stumbling Block Detox outlined in the following steps. These are developed with Laura Pringle, a wonderful coach. If we really lean in to these steps, it can be life-changing.

1) Notice when you start to feel excessively emotional. If your heart begins racing in anger or the tears start to rise up, really take note.

2) Make yourself pause. Stop talking! Go to the bathroom, or excuse yourself if you need to, or at least take a sip of water if you're at a meeting or a dinner. Train yourself to take some deep breaths, putting your full attention on your breath and not the situation.

3) After you've paused for at least a few moments, go right to the facts of the present situation. As in, the waiter forgot to bring my water, and I asked four times already. Or, my boyfriend interrupted me in the middle of my story about my big presentation to ask about the laundry.

4) Ask yourself, "Why does this situation upset me so?" Which really means "What is the story I am telling myself right now?" It could be the story that everyone ignores you, or that you can't be accepted for being yourself. Sometimes it's hard to tell, but if you sit with the question, you're opening the door to start healing your deepest wounds and deep, limiting beliefs. Let yourself sit in that awareness. As you go back into the situation and life, contemplate what beliefs you are walking around in the world with. How do these beliefs affect your life? Deep down, we all want to be loved and seen for who we really are.

5) By using this process over time, it becomes easier to identify the negative stories we often tell ourselves. And the more we do the exercise, the better our understanding of our inner hurts and the deep beliefs we carry around with us that are *behind* the upsets and certain behaviors. This awareness is a huge step in moving toward letting them go, and the freedom and wholeness that is possible.

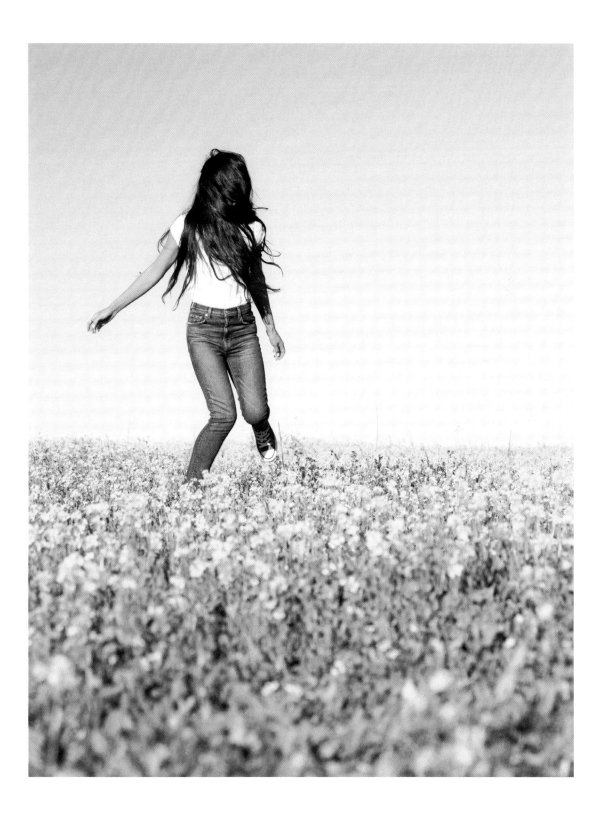

Curing Self-Judgment

Have you ever noticed how much judgment infiltrates conversations and the world around us? Instead of simply observing what we see in front of us, we often feel compelled to cast an opinion and verdict over it. Here are some examples:

Wow, that dress is really not very flattering on her. It makes her arms look huge!

She never cooks for her family. Isn't that so selfish?

His life is so unbalanced. It's all about his career, and he doesn't care about anything else.

She is so obsessed with herself. I can't believe how many selfies she posts.

That couple is so clueless about what is actually healthy. They say they are "into" wellness, but did you see what they ate at dinner?

You might hear, or say, such comments casually throughout your whole day—at brunch, in a moms' group, at work, or on talk shows and morning programs. When we tune in to judgment, we will see that it is pretty much everywhere. And we've all had our share of participating in it, too.

A few years ago, I was complaining to my friend Justin about a trip I had recently taken. I was staying with some acquaintances and it was a difficult experience. These people were so controlling! I felt like I had been interrogated with fifty questions in a row and was being judged left and right. Justin said to me, "You must have that same trait in yourself, and that's why they bug you so much."

At first I balked at the idea and vehemently denied that could be a possibility. I couldn't fathom at that point that I might actually be *like* these people. Yet deep

down, this provoking idea hit a nerve. And when I really peered inside myself, I could see that I, too, sometimes try to control situations by repeating myself over and over again, instead of trusting I was heard the first time.

life detox recipe

Pay attention whenever judgment comes up, as it can be a great teacher for us and a mirror for what we don't like in ourselves. Get a "judgment journal" and write out what you don't like in others. It could be pettiness, materialism, selfishness, being unfriendly, flaky, fake, or whatever. Spend some quiet time examining where you might have exhibited such traits in your own life—without feeling guilty. We're *all* struggling on our paths in some way or another. See what you can learn and where the roots of such traits may come from, such as coping mechanisms for not feeling good enough. Dedicated writing and reflection can help heal.

Psychoanalyst Carl Jung taught that we all have an unconscious drive to move toward wholeness and realization of the self. According to Jung, contained in our unconscious is our "shadow," which is the repressed thoughts, feelings, and ideas about ourselves that we push down rather than confront. Our judgment of others is a way of acknowledging disowned traits and behaviors within ourselves without having to face the pain of knowing the imbalance is actually within us. It's often agonizing for us to admit qualities or parts of us that we don't like, so our minds project outward and pick up these very qualities in other people.

We are not inherently negative or bad. Don't believe that for even a second! Yet we all do have areas for improvement. This isn't possible until we first see and admit that the qualities we gripe about in others (being catty, self-centered, moody . . . you fill in the blank!) can also exist within us. Of course, we may not express the quality in the same exact way. Let's say you find a coworker narcissistic; she always brings up personal stories at staff meetings. If you get annoyed in the moment and then let it go, that's natural. Yet if you become obsessed with someone else's flaws and then feel the need to gossip and comment about it any chance you can, that's an issue. Let's turn it around. How might you be narcissistic? Sure, you might not talk about yourself at staff meetings, but perhaps you talk on and on with your parents about your life and never ask them about theirs. Or maybe you always insist on eating at your favorite restaurants over those that your friends prefer.

I know looking at this stuff can be really hard for some of us! So why deal with the pain? Because as Jung would say, when we bring "our shadow into the conscious," it starts to lose power. And as it loses power, negative patterns of reacting melt away.

Start to notice when even a twinge of judgment comes to mind or out of your mouth. Whenever we are strongly critical of others' bodies, weight, skin, and other aspects of physical appearance, achievements, work, parenting, and so on, we are the most disapproving of *ourselves*. Check in with yourself. Judgment does not feel good, so pay attention to changes in the way you feel physically. Maybe you routinely experience a hollow feeling in your gut or even a dull ache around your chest or heart area. Start to tune in with the signals your body is giving you.

The cures for judgment are self-acceptance and living from a place centered on kindness and compassion for ourselves and others. When we open our hearts and stop judging ourselves, the need to judge others naturally drops away.

life detox recipe

Underneath, we all have traits that we don't care to acknowledge. The only way to bring those parts of us back into balance is to accept that they exist. This is painful for all of us, yet it's so worth the effort in order to feel more whole and happy. Eating cleansing foods to clear your system is very helpful for this. Toxicity creates stagnation that can block us physically, and it can also produce mental blocks (like moodiness and negative feelings), as the brain-gut axis links the health of our gastrointestinal (GI) tracts and how we feel.

Try recipes that are high in cleansing fiber and liver-supporting enzymes, since your liver is your main detoxifying organ and there is a connection between your liver and gut function.

Here are some great recipes for this:

» The JAPANESE SUPER-CLEANSE SALAD (page 121) contains fibrous cabbage and radicchio. Cabbage is a detoxifying cruciferous vegetable. A 2014 study published in the *Asian Pacific Journal of Cancer Prevention* suggests that cabbage is a source of important antioxidant and anti-inflammatory properties. The fresh lime in this salad is a natural diuretic and works to cleanse toxins from the body.

» The LIGHTNESS GREEN CUKE ROLLS (page 144) are based on ultra-hydrating cucumbers, which have lipid-lowering, antioxidant, and detoxifying properties. The avocado and basil sauce is fresh and full of fiber and water for easier digestion. The lemon juice helps to support the liver.

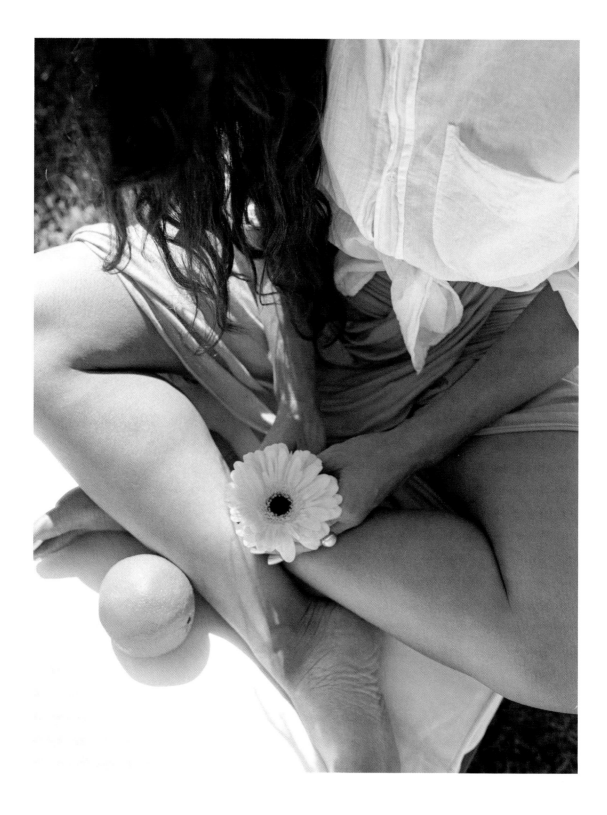

CHAPTER 3

(truly) loving our bodily temples

Letting Go of Bloating—and Letting Go in Life

We've all heard of the concept of letting go. Take the food that we eat. We need to chew it, digest it, process it, and then let it pass. If we hold on to it, it leads to bloating, which can lead to constipation, which can then lead to dangerous blockages in our digestive system. If we feel guilty about the food we eat and mentally reprimand ourselves for being "weak" for caving and eating deep-dish pizza or an extra slice of birthday cake, those feelings, emotions, and insecurities can further contribute to stress and poor digestion. When we hold on to things, we not only feel heavy and blocked, but we can make ourselves sick.

More and more scientific research is backing up the connection between our emotions and physical health. A study published in the *Journal of Physiology and Pharmacology* found that stress alters the brain-gut interactions ("brain-gut axis"), ultimately leading to the development of gastrointestinal disorders such as inflammatory bowel disease (IBD) and irritable bowel syndrome (IBS), in both of which bloating can be a symptom. Other studies suggest that cognitive behavioral therapy, hypnotherapy, and mindfulness-based therapy combined with conventional medical treatment helped to treat IBS better than conventional medical treatment alone. Moreover, these emotional and psychological practices helped calm patients' nervous systems and reduced inflammation. Clearly, our emotions and feelings do have considerable impact on the amount

life detox recipe

"Letting go" is a concept we can start to apply right away to our physical bodies, which helps us let go emotionally. Have you ever noticed that when you did a detox program or cleanse, you ended up cleaning out your closet or kitchen pantry? Detoxing one part of our lives helps other parts cleanse as well.

» To start "letting go" more, replace "sticky," congestive foods with ones that are more digestible. One example is replacing wheat bread or pasta with varieties based on quinoa, brown rice, lentils, or teff. Wheat, as well as barley and rye, contains gluten, a protein that many people have difficulty digesting, and also fructans, the carbohydrate compound that some newer research is finding might be the actual culprit within wheat that is responsible for irritable bowel syndrome.

» Check out the delicious LET GO GLUTEN-FREE PASTA WITH AVOCADO PESTO (page 190), which has a nonbloating, properly food combined pesto sauce based on avocado instead of nuts. (See page 84 for more information on the concept of *properly food combined*.) You can find pastas at health markets or online that are made with lentils, brown rice, and quinoa instead of wheat flour.

» Another congestive food to let go of is dairy. Since dairy is not created to be digested by the human body— it is created to nourish a baby cow—it is mucus- and acid-forming in humans, and some research has linked it with acne. Moreover, dairy is not a good source of absorbable calcium, despite what we may have been led to believe by the dairy industry and milk campaigns. The issue with dairy is that while it does supply calcium, it is acid-forming upon digestion, so the body has to neutralize that acidity by leaching alkaline minerals, namely calcium, which leads to urinary calcium excretion and an actual net loss of calcium. Harvard's Nurses' Health Study followed more than seventy-two thousand women for eighteen years, and its results showed that there was no protective effect of increased milk consumption on fracture risk.

» Try the TEMPEH TACO "MEAT" SALAD WITH CASHEW SOUR CREAM (page 118), which demonstrates how delicious nondairy cheeses and recipes can be, while leaving you—and your belly—happy!

» Letting go, going-to-the-bathroom-wise, is also key! Try taking oxygen paired with magnesium, which is a non-habit-forming way to cleanse waste more effectively from our systems without laxatives. It's really not just about eating well, but also cleansing out efficiently and as much as possible on an ongoing basis that makes an enormous difference in our energy, moods, health, skin, and ability to radiate and glow. See my website for a supplement called Detoxy, which is a powerful support for this.

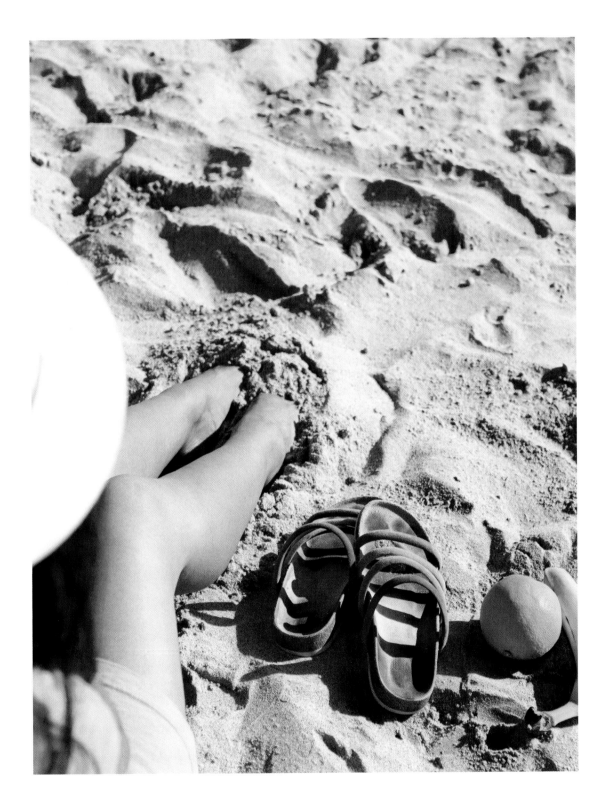

of physical and even spiritual bloating in our lives!

A client of mine, whom I will refer to as Melanie, is stunningly beautiful and talented in her craft. Yet she is constantly and painfully bloated nearly every day. Though everyone tells her how gorgeous she is, she tells me it is painful for her to look in the mirror! *Insecure* isn't a strong enough word. Melanie held on to a lot of childhood trauma and guilt, as well as a complex mother-daughter relationship that she hadn't processed. How could you tell? Because Melanie constantly commented about painful experiences she had growing up. The past was very much a part of her present day-to-day life. No matter how many food adjustments we made, probiotics and other digestive aids she took, or medical interventions and consultations with gastroenterologists she had, nothing seemed to improve her bloating in a long-term, substantial way.

Though I'm not a psychologist, I believe that her chronic bloating is in part related to holding on to her emotional blocks and wounds. Everything is connected to everything else, including our bodies and the thoughts in our minds and the feelings in our hearts (a concept that thankfully Western societies are finally starting to embrace!). Yet sadly, when I approached her with these ideas, she was unwilling to discuss this possibility further. As of the last time I spoke to her, she remains totally bloated.

When you hear the phrase *letting go*, what comes up? If you're like most of us, that Disney song might pop into your head. The idea of letting go in order to achieve happiness seems ubiquitous. But an idea without an action applied to it is really just about as dead a thing as there can be.

What are some things that you can let go of? Perhaps the rude comment from your aunt on Thanksgiving when she asked when you're going to "settle down." Maybe your colleague took credit for a project you did more work on. Maybe you're still thinking about a name someone called you when you were a child. Or maybe you can't let go of that idiot who looked your way and laughed when you messed up the moves at the dance cardio gym class. Silly as some of these might sound, emotional blockages can lead to what I like to call "irritable soul syndrome," which, in turn, can add to chronic bloating, IBS, constipation, or other forms of digestion issues.

life detox recipe

Sometimes we may subconsciously crave fatty and sugary treats, like ice cream, to shift our mood. It's okay to have treats here and there, though we don't want to get distracted from acknowledging the feelings at the same time. Choose noncongestive, properly food combined options so you avoid feeling sluggish. Don't worry—I have great dessert suggestions for you, including the two options below:

» The FUDGY CLEAN BLONDE BROWNIES (page 262), like all the recipes in this book, are gluten-free, plant-based, and properly food combined. They are sweetened with coconut sugar, which is a low-glycemic, low-fructose sweetener option that also contains trace minerals. In place of butter or oil, the recipe uses coconut oil, which is energizing and digests cleanly.

» The WHOLESOME BANANA CRISP (page 250) has a harder topping and a mushy middle—just like us! It's a great dessert to make and share (and enjoy) with loved ones.

The Letting Go technique, based on the process Dr. David Hawkins described in his book *Letting Go*, is to simply focus on fully experiencing our feelings, in order to let them go. To do so, it is necessary to pay

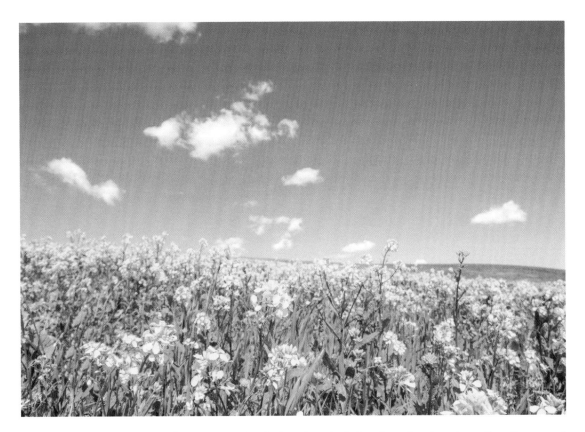

attention to any physical cues that come up. You don't have to name a feeling, as in "that is anger!" You can just feel the actual sensations that arise and be present to them, like an unsettled feeling in your stomach.

Focusing on the feeling itself, while often uncomfortable, can dissipate in around ten or so minutes. It doesn't usually last superlong if you focus only on the feeling itself. It doesn't feel great. In time, the feeling will cycle through and release from your body, like pulling out a giant weed from your vegetable garden. No questions, no wondering, no following thoughts. Simply sitting in it until it passes.

Emotional detox is just as important as paying attention to physical detox. Research has found that people with elevated levels of anxiety experience more gastro-intestinal disorders of various types than the general population.

Consider this: When you eat some fruit, you're getting water and nutrients and enzymes and calories and sugars . . . all things you need to keep you healthy and alive. Your body takes what's necessary and then expels what it doesn't need. Our minds and hearts should do the same. We can take something emotionally nutritious from an argument or a good or bad experience, take what's beneficial, and let the rest pass away from us. But we don't always do that. We hold on to past hurts that essentially change our DNA and our chemical makeup, which can eventually lead to disease.

When we take the good digestion approach to life, we start to see that even "bad" things can be beneficial and teach us valuable lessons. Someone may criticize you, or reject you, or you might get fired or rejected in an audition or job interview. See what you can learn and then let it go. As martial arts legend Bruce Lee used to say, take what helps you and discard the rest.

life detox recipe

As often as strong negative feelings arise—anger, anxiety, fear, and so on—apply the Letting Go technique described here. This is your continual plan for emotional detox. It does get easier, and eventually all the stored-up negative feelings start to empty out and take up less energy.

detoxing body shame

Body shame is a deep-rooted toxin that many of us carry. Statistics reveal that, even as children, we start to experience shame about our bodies, often because of what we've picked up from our parents and the adults around us. In fact, an online, nationally representative survey found that a whopping 94 percent of girls and 66 percent of boys had already experienced body shame by the time they became teenagers. Research on college women actually shows that shame can predict more poor health outcomes later, and negative body image is associated with depression, anxiety, and suicidal thoughts.

Body shame doesn't affect us just from a health and wellness perspective. It has been shown that girls with low body image tend to be less assertive, which can hold us women back professionally. It can also keep us from asking for the support we require and stating our needs, which are essential ingredients in the life recipe for feeling balanced and happy.

Most of us have been raised to feel that being heavy or overweight makes us less worthy, due to the societal prevalence of "antifat" attitudes. A 2014 survey reported that 85 percent of adolescents had observed overweight classmates being fat-shamed or teased in gym class. It's no wonder why we all too easily shame ourselves for gaining just a few pounds, or not being quite as thin as someone we happen to see on a social media hashtag! Weight discrimination, or fat shaming, has been shown to lead to declining physical and mental health over time. Imagine the detrimental, lifelong effects on your own health if you constantly shame yourself and your body.

Practicing compassion toward ourselves is a huge part of our own healing. We can know this on some level, yet harsh thoughts and judgments can easily slip in. Incorporating practices every day can help, as they support us in feeling consistently good from the inside. When you feel good, you're less likely to be mean to yourself.

Powerful practices I recommend include following a morning routine (outlined on page 25), taking some time to make nourishing recipes for yourself (such as the ones in Part II!), and practicing the kindergarten rule of saying something nice to yourself or nothing at all. The path to detoxing body shame is something we probably have to keep working on throughout our lives. We're all long-term works in progress together.

Our Amazing and Imperfect Bodies

How often do you look in the mirror and only notice how awesome your hair is, or how beautiful your smile is? How often do you take a moment to celebrate yourself and ignore any flaws and imperfections you see?

Probably not often . . . or never (especially if you just laughed out loud)! Most all of us pick at ourselves endlessly, seeing the zit that no one else does or the teeniest flyaway hair or bit of puffiness after a night of margaritas with friends. Modern researchers have now coined the phrase *compare and despair* to refer to contrasting ourselves with carefully constructed social media images and, in turn, ending up feeling bad about ourselves.

I've endured quite the battle with my own body image in the past. My biggest nemeses were my legs (I was obsessed with the width of my thigh gap) and my upper arms. I'd force myself to work out in ways I actually dreaded, such as pushing myself to run a certain number of minutes every day or dragging myself to a boot camp class. I would feel like crap and be moody if I didn't get to work out for "enough" minutes every day. I think it's safe to say that I didn't have a healthy mind-set.

Now, instead of staring at the mirror for an hour wondering if it looks like I have more cellulite on my thighs, I've learned to focus on the positives that stand

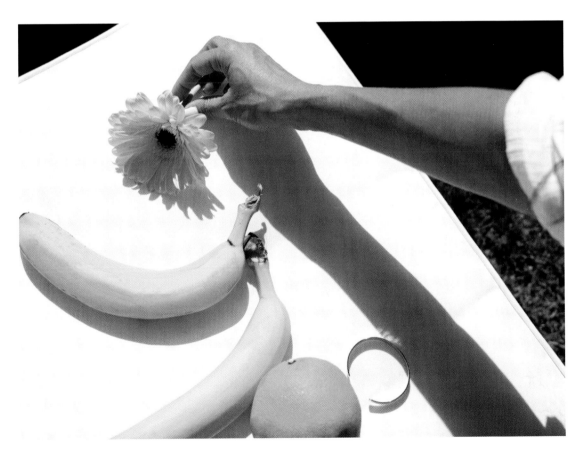

out to me about my body: I do like my thick, wavy hair (albeit the frizzy nest that it often is!), and I'm grateful that I like my hands and my stomach is strong and flat.

life detox recipe

True sexiness is a state of attraction we create from the inside, not something we paint on the outside.

To be truly sexy, we have to feel sexy, and this can be fostered by making wise choices for lunch. Eating a dense lunch, one that is overly oily, one full of processed deli meat and cheese, for instance, can make you feel heavy and stagnant for the rest of the afternoon or even the day. Not sexy. On the other hand, we don't want to skip lunch or eat a nutritionally defunct meal, as we need to support our vitality.

The key to lunch is choosing foods that give you long-sustaining energy and that contain fiber, as well as nutrients such as amino acids, antioxidants, B vitamins, vitamins A and C, and omega-3 fats.

Here are great lunch options I suggest:

» MINERALIZING ALMOND-GINGER KELP NOODLES (page 186).

» ENERGIZING PISTACHIO HEMPSEED CUCUMBER SALAD WITH ORANGE ZEST (page 115).

» NATURE'S COMPLETE PROTEIN SMOOTHIE (page 102), for a quick, light lunch on the go.

Yet this certainly was not my natural inclination. It took time and work to retrain my mind. There really isn't a magic pill you can take to suddenly feel total body acceptance. Change takes time, and some effort, yet it's a practice we can build on, like learning how to cook. Focus on small changes, then build from there. Train

yourself to focus your attention on three things you love about your body, and highlight them. For instance, if you love your legs, wear the pants or skirts that really show them off more often. If it's your eyes you want to emphasize, wear your hair back or in a way that frames them. To show off your smile, you can get a special lip gloss that makes you feel like a million bucks when you smile out in the world. This little bit of extra accentuation on the positive can build and expand the light of confidence.

I'm happy to say that I now only exercise in ways I absolutely love, which these days are mostly my barefoot beach walks, with the occasional hike with a friend and some yoga thrown in. I've had some really challenging times in the past few years, and I have found the beach walks keep me feeling the most grounded and centered.

I'm okay with my arms not being quite as strong as when I did dozens of daily *chaturangas* (a kind of yogic push-up) when I was doing more regular yoga asanas. And while my backside might certainly get more lift if I did some kind of barre class, I avoid such sessions because I personally don't enjoy them. Being happy and being outside are more important to me than a few inches of difference. Of course, some of us do enjoy such classes, or those few inches do make a big difference mentally. So there is no one way that is "right." It's all about being authentic to what feels good to you, versus being primarily motivated by running after approval or what other people think.

We all care about how we look, and that's just how it is. Yet we can also go beyond and connect deeply with our whole selves. Put your attention on how you *feel* in your body, and create practices and exercise routines that make you feel amazing—the healthy recipes in this book will certainly support that effort. You can focus on being in touch with your energy, strength, and intelligence (you fill in the qualities) and consciously direct your attention there so you don't fixate—and pick apart!—your outer appearance.

And you know what? As much as our society emphasizes perfect blowouts, toned abs, and flawless skin, nothing is more irresistibly attractive than being comfortable, happy, and feeling "good enough" just as you are. It's a magnetic energy that can't be bought. If you find yourself consumed with one little body flaw (as we *all* do sometimes), refocus on the three things you love about your body, and remind yourself that everyone in their own ways has a perfectly imperfect body, too.

life detox recipe

Daily practices anchor us to daily actions that leave us feeling great within our bodies. Here are a few practices I want to highlight:

MEDITATION. Starting and ending the day with even a few moments of conscious breathing can transform the day. It helps you feel present, which makes you feel good and powerful. Feeling scattered does not feel good. There are free guided meditations on my website if that would be helpful to you.

MIDMORNING PRACTICE. You might get hungry midmorning, depending on your activity level or constitution. It is so important at this point of the day to eat foods that support our energy, rather than deplete it. We often get hungry before lunch and we don't know what to eat! A common issue I see in my nutrition work is eating too-heavy foods at this time. The key is to stay away from foods that could interfere with digesting your lunch. Don't worry, I have great midmorning food options for you, including:

» The PINK ENERGY PORRIDGE (page 229) is made of energizing whole-grain or steel-cut oats and tart dried cranberries, which flush toxins from the body.

» The POWER PROTEIN BOWL (page 107) is particularly beneficial if you had a morning workout or need more fuel in the morning. The free-form amino acids of plant-based protein powders are a superior option, digesting well and without adding toxicity to your body. This recipe supplies about 20 grams of protein or more, depending on the type of protein powder you use and the granola you add on top.

EVENING COMEDOWN. Sipping something warm and comforting in the evening, while reading or relaxing, is a great ritual to prepare for rest time. Try the GINGER COMEDOWN HOT CHOCOLATE (page 267), which is creamy yet dairy-free and contains warming, metabolism-boosting ginger. If you feel really wound up, omit the cacao, which can be a bit stimulating for some, and follow the rest of the recipe, with the ginger slices, cinnamon, and so on.

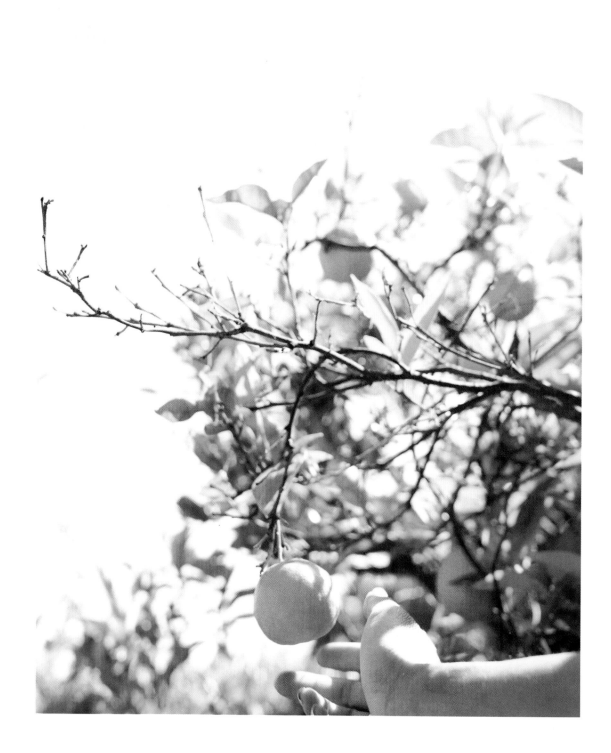

When Eating Gets Disordered

This is going to sound weird, but imagine your relationship with food as if it were a relationship with a person. Would you want to be involved with someone if your interactions were based upon rewards or punishments, indulgences and fasts? For many of us, our relationship with food mirrors a toxic relationship with another person.

On some level, many of us reading this right now have at some point had a warped relationship with food—from being a chocoholic or chronic yo-yo fad dieter or calorie slasher to having a raging sweet tooth (all these categories I have personally been in myself). And when our unhealthy food relationship becomes more extreme, it crosses into the spectrum of eating disorders. And in that realm, many of us have also struggled.

According to the National Association of Eating Disorders, more than ten million Americans report symptoms of an eating disorder, such as anorexia nervosa or bulimia nervosa. Many more might struggle secretly with these disorders, and millions more battle with binge-eating disorders. This all adds up to gigantic numbers worldwide.

My client, whom we'll call Maureen, was completely fixated on controlling the food in her life. Soon after we started working together, she was not comfortable eating anything until she described the food in detail (exact amount, seasonings, and so on) and, via text or a call, I gave my "approval" to eat it. It didn't really matter anyway, because she admitted that she would never eat all that I prescribed for her. She always had some excuse not to eat the substantial foods, claiming she felt nauseous or disliked the taste. To my great concern, Maureen would often eat just large amounts of the Probiotic and Enzyme Salad (raw sauerkraut) I made and other foods she knew had very few calories.

She was so thin, yet she complained about how big her belly and legs were. Eventually, it became clear to me that Maureen had an eating disorder, and she needed specialized, professional help.

life detox recipe

Besides our diets, loving self-care practices include meditation, making time for self-reflection, journaling, and (one of my personal favorites) walking and spending shoe-free time in nature. This last one makes us feel energized, connected to nature and the bigger whole, at the same time that it helps us feel expansive and free from the binds of obsession over body image.

Grounding or earthing—which is simply when we directly touch the earth, barefoot—puts us in sync with the earth's energy field and is electrically conductive, neutralizing inflammation-causing free radicals. It has been shown to be beneficial not only for the heart but also for reducing stress and increasing circulation and blood flow.

When I approached her about treatment, she denied needing it. I then brought it up to her manager, who agreed to do an intervention with me to get her professional help. It worked. Our relationship shifted. Instead of giving her constant reassurance and unknowingly enabling her to continue in her patterns, I was now there to give her love and support. Sometimes this meant challenging her. She knew that she needed to face her body image problem and rethink the way she treated herself. This wasn't always easy, and there were times when she felt I had violated her trust by initiating the intervention. Still, we work together, and while we're no longer in contact on a daily basis, we check in at regular intervals. She now closely follows my wellness program for her overall health, including drinking the Glowing Green Smoothie and doing my meditations.

I've had many readers share with me the stories of their eating disorders. I always encourage them to get professional help immediately and commit to the long journey toward choosing to love and accept themselves. Research has linked eating disorders to psychological traits such as low self-esteem, feelings of inadequacy or lack of control in life, depression, anxiety, anger, stress, or loneliness, which is why focusing seriously on fostering self-love is vital.

I learned this the hard way. In high school, I suffered for a time with a level of anorexia, as well as bulimia. I was so self-conscious that I mentally attacked myself daily for not being skinny enough every time I looked in the mirror. Even though I was five foot four and my weight at times was as low as ninety-five pounds, I constantly compared myself to images in ads and magazines and hated myself for being "fat." During that time I was obsessed with running and controlling what I ate. Yet I eventually became so hungry from all the running that I needed to increase my calories, which, to say the least, freaked me out. I resorted to purging for a time, which I hid from my family and everyone else. Those were dark, lonely times.

Part of my journey of healing entailed swinging to the other extreme before finding balance. I let go so much that when I got to college, I ate whenever and whatever I felt like, drinking loads of beer and vodka-based cocktails and inhaling late-night pizza. I stashed a supersize container of sugary animal crackers from Costco on the bookshelf in my dorm room and grabbed handfuls of them multiple times a day on the way to and from class. Fluffy white ciabatta bread sandwiches stuffed with cheese and hummus were a daily staple. I also ate french fries multiple times a week.

Going overboard with food was a welcome phase of relaxation from the extreme control I had previously imposed on myself. I might have started off slightly underweight, yet by the end of college I had gained quite a bit of weight and was on the heavier side. Another period of my body adventure began, which was experimenting with all different diets—even a brief foray with Atkins! And eventually, as the rest of the story goes in *The Beauty Detox Solution*, I learned how to truly find balance and heal my digestion and body.

We all have scars from our past, particularly regarding how we've abused our bodies and beat ourselves up mentally. For many of us women, some of those scars include our own versions of deep body shame (see page 44), self-hatred, and using tons of our energy dieting to try to be "good enough." Often, the inner scars hurt more than the outer ones.

What is the cure? Love. Choosing to love ourselves. It sounds basic, and we've heard it a million times before, but now we can focus on developing it from a new, powerful angle with some of the food and other suggestions throughout this book. We might have picked up some beliefs that we're not enough as we are, or that we are not lovable, and so we have to change ourselves or lose weight or look younger to be worthy, but none of these things are actually true. We don't *need* anyone else to love us in order for us to be "okay," though it's certainly nice to share life (and love) with others. The difference is the desperation. That love we are desperately seeking can come from our own selves.

A lack of self-love is the unnourished root of body shame, guilt, and unhealthy obsessions. The end goal is not about eating only the right foods or getting optimal nutrition, or reaching the ideal weight. We can have a "perfect" body and still hate ourselves. Being healthy and happy and truly well is centered in us being more soft and gentle with ourselves. We can start to *experience* that we are so much more than a number on a scale or the outer shell that is the shape of our bodies.

Healing our relationship with food, in parallel to healing our relationship with ourselves, takes time, effort, patience, and great compassion. Like any relationship, there are periods where it seems easier to get along, and sometimes it's so hard we want to break down and cry. Yet each tiny, growing awareness, each time we reflect and are a little kinder with ourselves, and each healthy recipe we choose to make and nourish ourselves with is a step closer to discovering healthiness with food and ourselves.

life recipe

Home-cooked meals are a powerful way to love and give energy back to yourself. When we pick up processed fast foods to eat all the time, it may be convenient, but they're devoid of vitality. Just really look at it next time it comes in your space! It doesn't look like very "happy" food, made lovingly or with care, does it? It feels thrown together, made in mass, and, to be frank, a bit sad. By putting it in our bodies, we send ourselves the message on some level that we aren't worth the time to make real food.

I know, I know—you get it, but you're so busy. And after a long day at work or with the kids, the last thing you want to do is crack out your apron and prepare for a full-on kitchen session. So, how do we incorporate home cooking when we all live crazy, busy lives? With crazy, easy food! Simple can be really tasty and doable. Check these recipes out:

» GINGERY BASIL TEMPEH AND SNAP PEAS (page 180) can be made in five to ten minutes (depending on how fast you can chop!). It's packed with mineral- and nutrient-dense veggies and fantastically protein-rich non-GMO tempeh.

» EASY PROTEIN SAGE GARBANZOS (page 206), served with a quick-tossed salad, is another superfast nurturing meal. It's full of cleansing radishes and protein, vitamin C, antioxidants, and calcium from the kale.

» Check out the delicious and easy CUMIN ROASTED BRUSSELS SPROUTS WITH QUINOA (page 194), another powerful protein- and mineral-packed meal. I recommend batch-cooking more quinoa than you need for this recipe; it's a great way to have an excellent staple ingredient to toss in with easy recipes or to simply eat alongside salads.

» Throwing food in the oven so you are free to do other things is a great strategy for busy people cooking at home. You can make a big dish of the BOUNTY EARTH SALAD (page 130), cooking the root veggies in the oven while you change or shower or relax, and you'll have some delicious leftovers to bring to work for a few days.

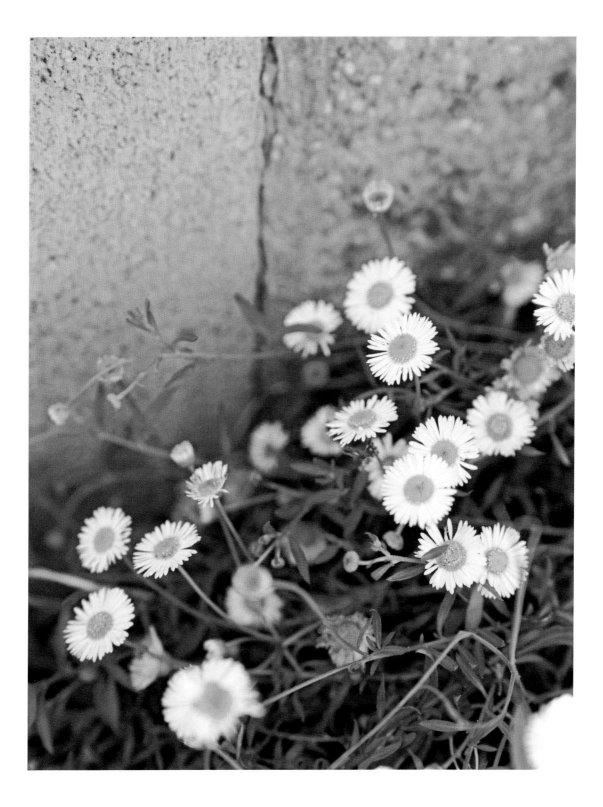

Going Not So According to Plan

I'm sure you've heard the old adage "People make plans, and God laughs." Isn't that the truth! Life can just push our buttons. We may make the best plans only to have them fall apart right before our very eyes.

This is exactly what happened to me with the birth of my son, Emerson—or Lil' Bub, his nickname. I fully intended to have a "natural" birth, meaning vaginally and without any Western medical interventions, at home.

Fast-forward several months. Bub's due date came and went. A checkup with Dr. Chin, my backup Western doctor, measured the baby close to a whopping nine pounds. Both Dr. Chin and my midwife were very concerned about the baby's large size fitting through my particular body and pelvis, and serious potential issues like shoulder dystocia and maternal hemorrhaging. But I insisted on sticking to my idea of the perfect "natural" birth.

After another week, with Bubby getting bigger by the day, my water broke in a huge gush during a midnight trip to the bathroom. Contractions started afterward but were not yet superclose together. I had been warned by my midwife that once my water broke, I had only twenty-four hours to go into active labor at home, defined as contractions coming three minutes or less apart, before I would have to be transported to the hospital because of possible risk of infection. So I went into somewhat of a panic, thinking, *Crap! Only about eighteen hours to accomplish my perfect birth!*

Instead of resting at home, I decided I should *do* as much as possible. I rushed to an acupuncturist specializing in "speeding up" labor. I drank nearly half a bottle of castor oil—something so foul I gag even as I write this. I started pumping with a breast pump, trying to push the contractions—which were still superintense, by the way—closer together.

No matter what I did, the twenty-four-hour time limit passed without the contractions speeding up enough, and there was no choice but to go to the hospital. The home-birth option had vanished. I brightened when my midwife insisted I could still have a beautiful "natural" birth at the hospital. *Ah, all is not lost!*

life detox recipe

Our lessons in life are unique, and so is our way of getting there. One way is not "better" than another. Sometimes we go a way that significantly shifts from prior expectations or plans, and the more we trust life is bringing us where we need to be to grow, the more we can let go of trying to control everything and just enjoy the ride. Be sure to also honor this truth for others. Everyone is on a different journey, and we can't compare our paths to others' paths and judge them. It's better to compare ourselves to who we were yesterday than to compare ourselves to someone else who has had a different upbringing, support systems, and genetics and who is on a totally unique life journey. In yogic terms, we would say we all have different karma to work out.

Try to sit back and stay unattached to your opinions. They evolve as you evolve. Being open and flexible to new ideas and perspectives allows us to learn important lessons and increase our wisdom.

But after hours of labor at the hospital, I had dilated all the way, yet Bubs still hadn't arrived. Things started to become precarious. My midwife thought I would "feel" the pushes more if I was given a very high dosage of Pitocin—with no epidural. I was groggy from the exhaustion and pain, and remember being unsure what was right at that point. Was this still going to be "natural" if I was starting to get drugs?

The next two hours were pure hell. There was a physical trauma of pain that I had never before experienced. These were certainly not "natural" contractions. They were strongly augmented Pitocin contractions, with no epidural or anything else to alleviate the pain. Now it had been four hours of pushing. Almost fifty total hours of labor.

It was at that point Dr. Chin strode back into the room and announced, "I can't allow this to go on anymore. This is a square peg in a round hole. The baby isn't coming out this way. I've let you try for as long as I think it is safe."

There was only one thing left to do: Cesarean section. It was like a strange dream. What started as a home birth was now ending in C-section. But I could not have been more relieved at that point. *My baby was coming to me, safely!* That was all I cared about, and all the focus on defining "natural" was gone in an instant. Who cared how the baby was born, as long as he was safe? And an epidural! Praise the Lord! I was elated to accept it.

By the way, my mother, sister, cousins, and aunt have all had C-sections. That side of the family hails from

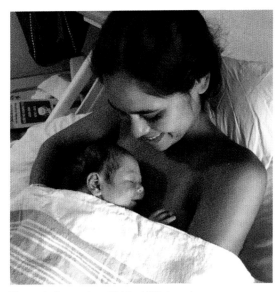

The magical, crazy, beautiful day Lil' Bub was born.

the Philippines, and like me, they have pretty narrow pelvises. Sure, my grandmother had natural births, but my Filipino grandfather is a lot smaller than the larger Caucasian men that all the other women in the family ended up having babies with. Yet these are all facts I chose to ignore because I insisted on sticking to *the* one-and-only plan.

The C-section was wonderful. Bubby came out smoothly, crying and full of life. After a few quick moments, he was put directly on my chest, skin to skin, where he stayed from then on (for pretty much the entire first year of his life!) and suckled up my colostrum.

Geez. As you can see, I really built something up only to have it fall apart. This is something we can *all* relate to. Maybe you thought a relationship was going to be "it," and you started looking at wedding dresses online, only to discover a few weeks later that your mate was nowhere near being ready to commit. Or perhaps you banked on the perfect yoga retreat to Bali to relieve all your pent-up stress, and it turned out you booked it during a monsoon and ended up being stuck in your hotel room–alone—most of the time. How can we best handle whatever happens in our lives?

One of the greatest things we can do is to let go of thinking it has to be or look a certain expected way, and to release labels, such as "good" and "bad"—however those terms are defined, anyway.

What if we started trusting that our lives are about growth, and that in some way, life is bringing us what we need to grow? Can we let go of attachments and expectations, which set us up for misery? Because if things don't pan out exactly that way, we think it's all bad and terrible. And we lose out on a chance for freedom, which is being able to feel joyful in any circumstance.

In Buddhism the concept of nonattachment refers to

life detox recipe

Expect life to work with you, but when it doesn't, expect to work with it. We can lay out the best plans and intentions, but the flow of life might have other designs for us. Flexibility and open-mindedness are important qualities to foster, and incorporating foods that encourage fluidity rather than rigidity in our joints and throughout all of our organs and tissues is a powerful way to manifest this quality in our lives now.

The right fats are key for optimal fluidity. We want to make sure to consume more plant foods that are rich in omega-3-fats, which include chia, flax-, and hempseeds; dark, leafy greens and weeds; Brussels sprouts; cauliflower; and so on. These wonderful foods help keep our bodies supple. And while fish also contains omega-3 fats, I recommend avoiding consuming it because of heavy metal exposure and also for environmental reasons; fishing is responsible for millions of sharks, dolphins, turtles, and other beautiful ocean life being killed in nets. At the same time, we want to reduce overconsumption of omega-6-containing foods, such as junk foods that contain loads of vegetable oil, which creates inflammation. Other fats to avoid include rancid or fried fats, and excessive saturated fats from meat and poultry.

Here are some great recipes to support flexibility and fluidity:

» The I WANT IT ALL SMOOTHIE (page 105) includes CHIA GEL (chia seeds soaked in water; page 104). Chia seeds are an excellent source of omega-3 fats, as well as cleansing fiber, antioxidants, amino acids, and minerals.

» The OMEGA-ARUGULA SALAD WITH PECANS AND LIME VINAIGRETTE (page 124) contains flax oil, which is another great source of omega-3 fats. Remember to refrigerated flax oil and never heat it, in order to retain its integrity. Arugula is a cleansing bitter green that detoxifies the blood of wastes.

» Speaking of oils, you will see that in all our baked desserts in this book, including the delectable DOUBLE CHOCOLATE CHIP AND OATMEAL COOKIES (page 266), we bake only with coconut oil. Coconut oil has a high smoke point, meaning it maintains its structure during cooking and doesn't become rancid. It is more easily burned off as energy instead of being stored as fat or congesting our bodies. I do not recommend baking with vegetable-oil- or plant-based butters, dairy products, or most other oils.

» STRENGTHENING WARM BOK CHOY WITH ROSEMARY DRESSING (page 149) contains loads of bioavailable calcium, and it also encourages fluid yet strong movement and structure to our bones and bodies.

---

the idea of surrender. No matter what comes our way, we can be centered and ultimately okay with it. We start to know that the source of joy and contentment is within us, not from the outside relationships or job or validation or likes on our social media posts. We can avoid suffering by surrendering to whatever comes. And by giving up the rigid labels of "bad" and "good" to accept simply what *is*.

This is far different from how most of us look at the world and our lives. Yet it is a powerfully liberating perspective that you can apply to your life, starting today.

Practice surrender with little things, such as altering some weekend plans because of the weather or choosing a different restaurant because your first choice is full. As you practice it and it feels good, it will help you out in more momentous situations, such as not getting the job after three interviews. Or accepting that a relationship wasn't meant to last as you go through a painful divorce. Nonattachment builds like a muscle: the more we practice it, the stronger we get. And our strength can ultimately carry us through anything.

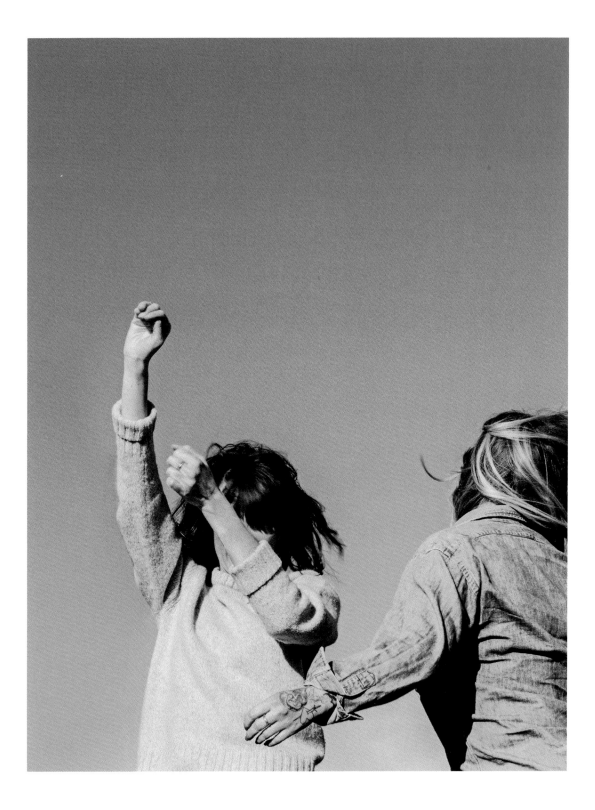

raising our vibration

Beauty Scars

As we've already discussed, life is unpredictable. Try as we might, we aren't in control of everything. Things often happen that we wish hadn't: a sudden breakup, a friend moves to another state, an injury while skiing, or events from our childhood that still bring a tear to our eyes.

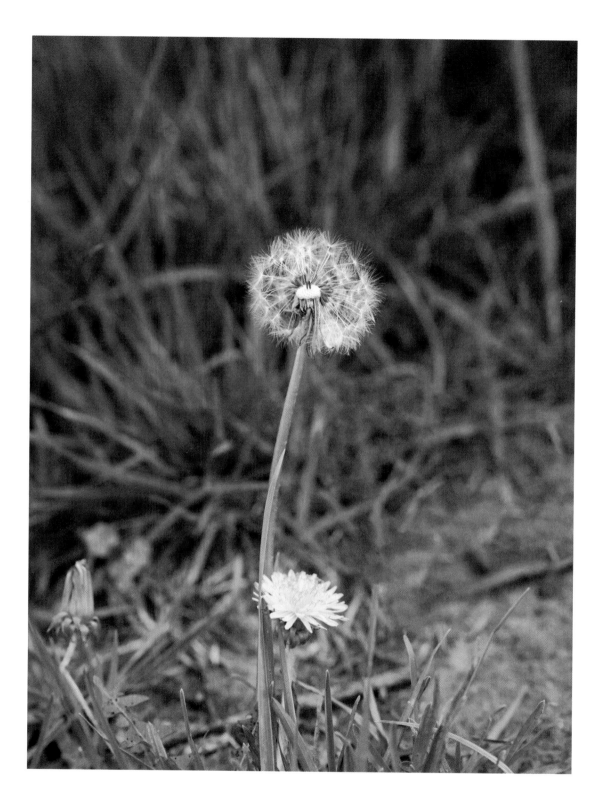

It's natural to want to avoid pain and heartache. It hurts! Yet when we stop wishing something had not happened to us and accept that it did, we can start digesting the lessons from it and find the gifts.

So, where are these so-called gifts? Sometimes we may want to shout: *Where ARE the freaking gifts!* From our current perspective, it just doesn't seem fair, it doesn't make sense, or it just isn't right. When my mom was diagnosed with cancer, I was shocked and terrified, but quickly rallied by her side, trying to support her in every way I knew how. I was convinced she was going to recover. She was so strong. Yet within six quick weeks when it became clear that my mom was not going to get better, I had to process deep sadness and resentment that I was losing her in my life far earlier than I ever thought I would—and before Bubby was even a year old.

Emotional pain often occurs when we resist what is. We're all going to feel stings and indescribably deep hurt when something initially happens, but after a length of processing or grieving time, if we don't work toward acceptance, and if we continue to feel angry or depressed, we hold on to that unprocessed energy, and it creates toxic psychological and spiritual blocks. In contrast, when we can survive the deepest pain and make it to the other side, then we truly realize how strong we are.

Imagine you are sitting on the beach at the edge of the water daydreaming, unaware that a huge wave is approaching. Then, crash! It hits you like a ton of bricks and tosses you back. After the wave passes, as you sit

life detox recipe

If you are moving through processing and letting go of something that causes pain for you, there are helpful foods that can start to enact that energy on the physical level, which will translate psychologically, emotionally, and spiritually. Here are some excellent ones to call out:

» GOJI BERRIES. This is a stabilizing food that supports our vitality and true beauty. Gojis are a rich source of antioxidants that protect our bodies from inflammation and fortify our immunity. They are full of vitamins and contain eighteen different amino acids that keep us grounded while walking through the fire. Try the GOJI BERRY SOOTHE BARS (page 248).

» SPROUTS + BITTER GREENS COMBO. Healing and detoxifying emotional blocks requires change, and enzymes are the dynamic entities that catalyze biological reactions. Sprouts are baby plants in the process of maturing, and they are bursting with enzymes and numerous other micronutrients. Bitter greens are cleansing and detoxifying, and help clear the way for more regeneration. The GREEN POWER SPROUT SALAD WITH CREAMY CITRUS DRESSING (page 116) is perfect for this. Use arugula as the green base. Along these lines, digestive enzymes are an excellent idea to take before meals, to help promote breaking down and optimal assimilation of key nutrients (see my website for more information).

» TURMERIC + ROOT VEGETABLE COMBO. The herb turmeric has received a lot of play in the media lately as a potent anti-inflammatory and cleansing food, even though it has been used in Ayurveda for over five thousand years. Here we are talking about more deeply integrating change, so I like to combine turmeric, which is detoxifying for your blood and therefore your entire body, with root vegetables, which provide an earthy, steadying, grounding element to hold the space for the integration. The SWEET CLEANSE TURMERIC-ROASTED ROOT VEGGIES (page 136) is exactly suited for this purpose.

there in the wake, you can stew in anger, which devital- izes your organs and creates inflammation and adrenal exhaustion, and feel wretched, or you can accept that now you are wet but you're still breathing! Maybe even in this awareness you giggle because you realize you were fantasizing and not paying attention to the fact that you were on the edge of the shore and waves are going to do what waves are going to do. Now you can start to wonder, *What did I learn from this experience—that I can survive and be okay even if I get knocked down unexpectedly? Also, can I find more humor and not take life so seriously?* If we are committed to shifting our compass toward finding the gifts, find them we will.

A client of mine, whom we'll call Audrey, grew up watching her father hit her mother. Then when Audrey was five, he left them and cut off all contact. Her mom worked double shifts as a cleaning lady to support them

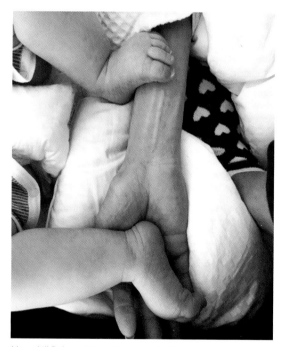

Mom, Lil' Bub, and I together in the final weeks.

both. Audrey never fully processed this formative part of her life, and to this day she has had difficulty trusting men. She self-sabotages every relationship she has, even if it's with a man who genuinely loves and cares for her. She admitted to me that she still carries a lot of shame about not being able to protect her mother, though it logically doesn't compute, as she was only a child.

Pain in life can propel tremendous growth, once we let go of resentment. Harboring resentment is the result of believing that something or someone should be differ- ent than it is. So in other words, this bitterness is simply more resistance, more pain, and more trapped emotional toxicity that creates more work for us to detox later. That's a lot of "mores." Yet when we soften and let the hard edges of resentment melt—when we realize that what is hap- pening now *is* happening, that there is no alternative— we allow the healing to come with acceptance.

I have come to peace with my mom's passing, and to be honest, while I still miss her physical presence, the sound of her voice, the way she smiled when she held Lil' Bub, I feel more connected to her in some ways than I ever have before. While my life will never be the same now that she's gone, I have learned that love is everlast- ing, and I accept that it was her time to learn and grow somewhere else.

My mom's passing has also given me a new look on time. In Einstein's general theory of relativity, there's no conceptual distinction between the past and the future. Physicists like Julian Barbour, the author of *The End of Time*, promote "timeless physics." If such theories are true, it would mean that time isn't really linear, and we can heal past events in the present. While there is some- thing to be said for moving forward in life, processing and digesting the past is necessary to release it and clear space for new energy in the future.

We need not feel that we have to hide or be embarrassed or push down what we've been through, no matter what it is. We're here today, alive and standing. Yes, we've weathered some storms and perhaps lived through some nightmares. Yet we can move forward. We can find ways to learn and gain higher understanding. The scars we accumulate along the way are part of our paths and, therefore, our unique beauty.

Approval Addicts

Do you feel a tiny little thrill when you see that a bunch of random people liked your Instagram pic? Or when you get a compliment after you lose a few pounds or get a new haircut? The answer is . . . of course! We all like approval because it activates a primal desire and need for survival. Millions of years ago our ancient ancestors would shun members of their tribe who seemed to do something that could jeopardize the whole. This disapproval often meant death because it meant trying to survive in the harsh wilderness alone. So approval really boiled down to issues of safety and security, and that got hard-wired in us. We also now know that approval also helps release dopamine, the neurotransmitter that helps control the brain's reward and pleasure center.

The dark side of seeking approval is that when we experience disapproval, our self-image takes a nosedive. As discussed, we've been conditioned to attach approval to security from ancestral brain wiring, and also from parents when we are young or from peers when we are teens, so disapproval seems to threaten our sense of security. The slower-acting cortical neurotransmitters, including acetylcholine and norepinephrine, are modified in response to emotional reactions, so there is also a chemical reaction in our brains making us feel off and uneasy when we spend an hour writing a social media caption and no one comments, not even our best friends. Or our boss casually remarks that our hair looked better before our big new haircut, or our parents imply they wish we had a "better" job . . . or boyfriend. Since we can't control what others think of us, chasing self-worth from the approval of others can lead to us making safer choices or ones that don't feel totally natural to us, and is a turbulent roller-coaster of ups and downs. And that ride is no fun.

When we prioritize others accepting us over accepting ourselves, we tell ourselves that we need to be who *they* want us to be, not who we are. Think about that—that is just terrible! We can only be who we are. Otherwise, we lose sight of who we are in order to change ourselves for more likes or attention. Not only does this make us unhappy deep down, but others can sense it as a lack of stability and confidence, and feel that they can't really know or trust who we really are.

We can actually validate and approve of ourselves, so that we don't have to agonize over getting it from everyone else. We *can* feel amazing in our new outfit, regardless of whether anyone else comments on it. We can have a great time at the party, regardless of how many guys look at us (or not). What if we just really enjoyed the music and conversations? And what if we just had fun with social media, only posting what feels natural and good to us and not obsessing over the likes. I'm not saying it's easy, and I'm not saying I don't still struggle with it, because I do. Yet I know that the more connected we each feel to ourselves—and the deep core of truth, compassion, and love that is at the center of all of us—the better and more peaceful we feel. And the need for those thrill-based approvals from the outside world will start to diminish.

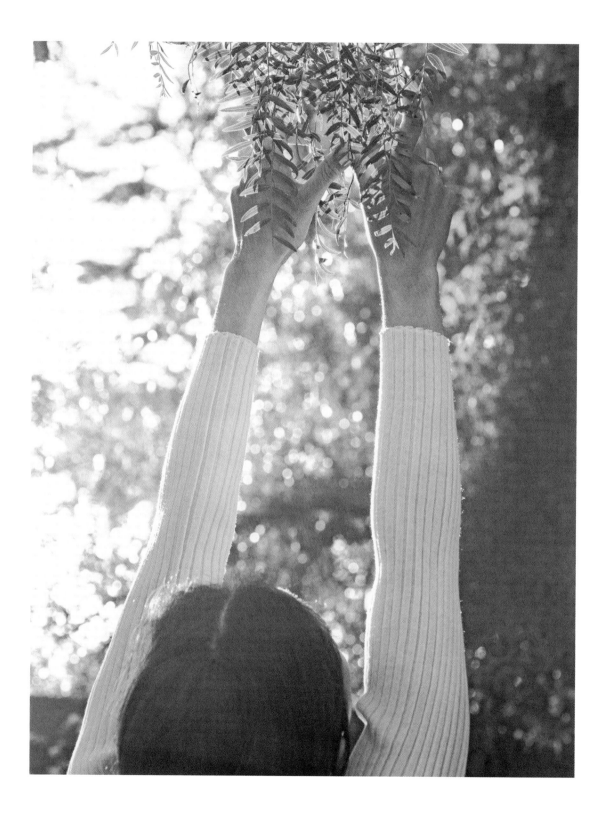

We discuss meditation and other stillness practices quite a bit, because they are *the* most powerful way I know to actually create and sustain happiness. It's like plugging into an energy socket that connects us to everyone and everything. When we move through life disconnected, we feel alone, small, weak, and depressed. Yet we always have access to the socket, which comes from tuning inward. If we keep practicing and persevering, especially with some definite techniques, then we can teach our noisy "monkey minds" to become quiet. We can learn to flood ourselves with peace and love, and we don't need a single other person to feel complete.

Creating the time to "plug in" and go within is essential to connecting to your wholeness. Without the stillness, we're left feeling more fragmented in the chaos of life. At first we may think distraction is better. It's fun and easy to call a friend or turn on the TV or watch a YouTube video or whatever. But eventually, that tiny distraction will wear off and there we are, as starved for approval as ever. The world will not give it to you, because the world is interested in making you feel you aren't enough and that you need to buy more stuff.

You can try any type of meditation practice that feels good to you (I offer some free meditations on my website, if that might be helpful to you), or just have some quiet time while driving, without chatting on the phone or blaring music. You can go for a walk by yourself, maybe listening to some wordless music or the birds or the rumblings of the urban space around you. Inner-stillness time can take many forms and look many different ways. Find the ones that resonate the most with you, and practice them. Plug in regularly, and stay charged.

life detox recipe

When we feel strong, nourished, and energized in our bodies, we can get plugged in much easier. It feels awesome. In contrast, if we are achy, gassy, bloated, belching, or feel downright heavy or gross in our bodies, such distractions make us feel . . . not so awesome.

Here are some great recipes to support you plugging into the source of everything magical and beautiful:

» The KALE, AVOCADO, AND GRAPEFRUIT SALAD (page 122) provides you with beauty fat; amino acids; vitamins A, C, and K; cleansing and detoxifying fiber; and so much more. You'll feel light and radiant as a rainbow after you eat this. Try it for lunch or as part of dinner to lay the foundation for a wonderful meditation a few hours later.

» CHICKPEA STEW WITH PISTACHIO PESTO (page 169). Stews are comforting soul food. Nuts are magical foods from Mother Nature that help us feel more grounded and stable and strong. After all, they contain the potential to grow into a mighty almond or walnut tree. This recipe is packed with minerals and protein to give you the stabilizing strength you need.

» MILLET MAGIC STUFFED 'SHROOMS! (page 197) supply you with protein- and vitamin-D-rich portobello mushrooms, as well as millet, which is really a superseed rich in protein and minerals, though we cook it like a grain.

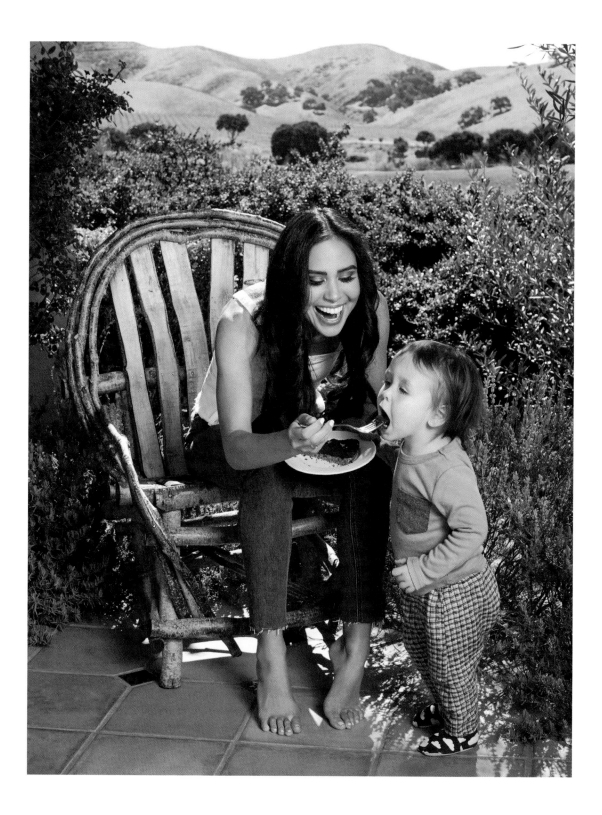

CHAPTER 5

happy, not perfect

Nope, I Don't Always Eat Perfectly

Sometimes, I really love soft, mushy tofu stir-fried with tamari (basically gluten-free soy sauce) and topped on a pile of rice. It kind of reminds me of the fried-egg-on-rice dish my mom and auntie would make me for breakfast when I was a kid. I don't eat eggs anymore, but I love that memory and the texture of the simple tofu dish that emulates it.

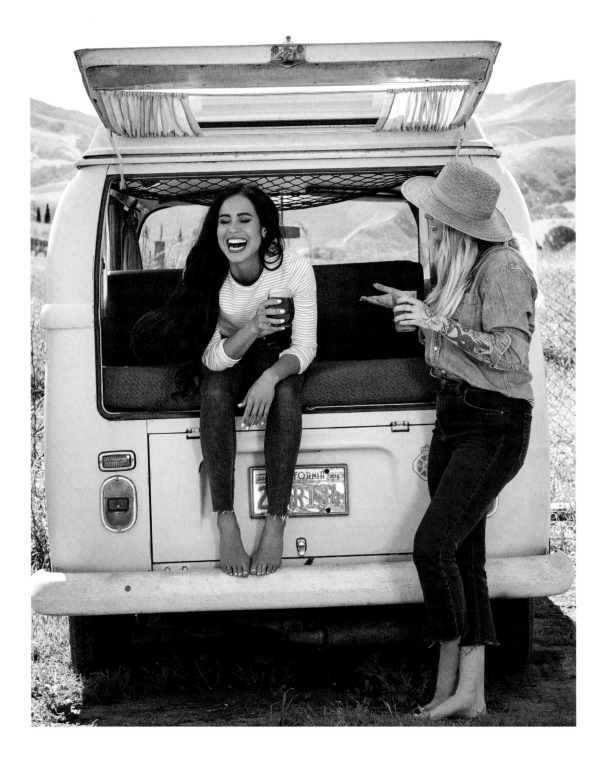

Wait, you might say (if you've read *The Beauty Detox Solution* or any of my articles on food combining; info also on page 84): Isn't tofu a protein and rice a starch? Isn't that bad food combining (gasp!)? Don't you write about avoiding that in your books?

Well, yes, it is improper food combining as a matter of fact! Yet I like the way it tastes, and I eat it sometimes. One of the biggest misconceptions that you might have about me is that I eat perfectly. I do not. A mantra of my philosophy is "Progress, not perfection." And I very much live by that, which is so important for recovering perfectionists like me.

It's not about trying to be at 100 percent, but striving for my 80/20 rule, or eating on track 80 percent of the time, and using that important 20 percent for favorite desserts, chips, and, yes, sometimes bad food combinations! And on occasion, especially when traveling, that 20 percent *does* stretch to a much higher percentage.

Do I have any guilt or shame or think I am a hypocrite because I write about food combining and don't *always* follow it? No. I'm a work in process, as we all are. We all do things we are less than proud of. Sometimes we do things we tell others not to do. We all slip. And it's okay, because it is our perfectly imperfect side shining through in all its flawed beauty.

life recipe

Perfection, especially in a dietary sense, is not the goal. Progress and overall consistency are. Trying to eat perfectly all the time is as rigid as walking on a tightrope, and it's a recipe for anxiety and unhappiness. Here are some great less-than-"perfect" comfort recipes to enjoy:

» I LOVE YOU FLATBREAD PIZZA (page 232). Okay, it is in the Kids' Corner chapter, but it is really for adults and children alike. My dad and other adult family members adore it! Plant-based commercial cheeses may be more processed, and they are certainly not right from the garden. They contain vegetable oils and other less-than-ideal ingredients, yet they are a pretty darn great option when we want a great dairy- and gluten-free pizza and/or are transitioning off dairy.

» MINT-CHOCOLATE LOVER'S BROWNIES (page 260). It is okay to indulge in chocolate sometimes (or every day, as I admittedly do in periods!), which does have some antioxidants—though we would eat it anyway without them, as it tastes so heavenly. And while we don't want to be sugar fiends, it's okay to have some sugar from time to time. Yes, it is okay! I know all the research points to how inflammatory and toxic sugar is. But life, and our diets, need room to be perfectly imperfect. And the sugar in this recipe comes from coconut sugar and coconut nectar, which are at least low glycemic and low fructose, and contain some minerals.

» COCONUT WOW COOKIES (page 259). This and the other baked recipes in this book were created after much trial and error, and by way of utilizing the special KS GLUTEN-FREE FLOUR MIX (page 252) that allows for the baked goods to bind, without egg or gluten, while also being properly food combined (see page 84). In our recipes, almond flour (a protein) is not combined with brown rice flour (a starch), for instance. Sure, we don't necessarily eat cookies every single day, but this is an amazing option for those occasions when we do want to!

We're All a Mess (At Least a Lot of the Time)

We're all messes in our own ways. We do our best, though we mess up left and right, and keep soldiering on. It's all good because messing up is how we test and retest the recipes of life and figure things out. Don't get me wrong, screwing up a recipe and having to start over from scratch isn't fun. Neither is sabotaging a relationship and having to put the pieces of your life back together in the aftermath. Yet, all of these mishaps are part of our grand unfolding journey toward peace and wholeness. If we didn't have these experiences, we wouldn't have any depth. We'd be stuck in the shallow, kiddy end of the pool, instead of braving the deeper, murky waters, which develops character, presence, and wisdom.

life detox recipe

When you mess up in the little things of life, laugh about it. Don't take it so seriously. Forget to do one task before a meeting and get called out . . . whoops! Remind yourself to be more thorough next time. Burn dinner . . . let out a good laugh and order Chinese food. If someone points out how you stumbled, see what—if anything— you can learn from a humble, nondefensive place.

When you value the wisdom of the bad days as much as the beauty of the good days, or the mess-ups as much as the smooth times, you will no longer need life to be any other way than it is.

I started going to Mommy and Me classes as a first-time mom when Lil' Bub was about eight weeks old, and I felt very self-conscious. Was I holding him right? Changing his diaper right? Did I have all the stuff in my diaper bag I was supposed to pack? Or was I utterly screwing up as a mom?

One day I got to class a bit late, and the class leader glanced over at me and, right in front of the circle of moms, said, "Your carrier isn't on right. Let me help!" I felt a flash of shame and thought, *Oh my gosh! I did it wrong, and I almost suffocated my baby!* Then I realized it was fine. Bub's head was up, and he was totally safe; the carrier was just a few inches off from where it should have been sitting on my waist. As I looked around while the group leader helped me adjust the straps, I could see that the other moms were focusing on their own mini-crises and babies. No one really cared.

The truth is people judge you. They just do. While we talked about working on not constantly casting judgment (see page 36), it's a lifelong practice. For all of us, some dialogue passes through our minds about people's voices or the way they look or how they act at a party or whatever.

But here's the kicker. Even though someone passes judgment on you, it usually doesn't last for a long time. Why? Because we all have other things on our minds. Maybe a mom looked at me when the instructor first mentioned my mistake and thought, *What a dummy!*

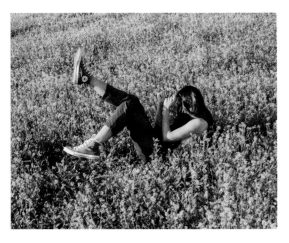

But then her mind quickly shifted to a bill she needed to pay or what she was going to make for dinner, and then her mind jumped again to the booger hanging from her baby's nose.

Even if fleeting comments crop up from others, who really gives a damn? Even when you totally mispronounce a word in a presentation, or totally botch up your latest relationship, or lose your temper with your friend at a party when you've had a little too much to drink . . . just clean up the mess, learn, and move on. We all screw up, but *we* are not screwups.

Guilt Cleanse

Melanie is a full-time consultant who has worked on some special projects for Solluna. She is also a mom of two. Working from home, she manages to excel in her projects, drive her son to and from preschool, and nurse her one-year-old (a nanny also helps during work hours). She cooks dinner for the family, and bedtime includes both of her kids piling into bed to sleep with her and her husband. Often, once they are asleep, she pulls out her laptop to get more work done. Yes, she is sort of a superhuman! Some time ago, when she came to LA to stay with me, she was flabbergasted when she saw me put nineteen-month-old Lil' Bub down at seven o'clock at night, leaving me the evening and the first part of the morning free and clear.

"I love having Bubby playing around me all day while I work. I take him in the stroller during conference calls, get a lot of writing done during nap time, and am beyond grateful I have my dad and auntie at home with us, which keeps the household from imploding. Yet, if I didn't have that 'me time' every day after he goes to bed in his own room, I think I'd lose my mind!" I told her.

life detox recipe

Make recipes that may or may not come out exactly right, and have fun with the results, no matter what they are. It's a good practice for dropping the superstressful "good/bad" labels in life, and working with whatever shows up.

» CRANBERRY CINNAMON MUFFINS (page 215). Sometimes muffins are a bit tricky. You might accidentally leave them in too long, and they dry out and harden. Or if they don't bake long enough, they totally stick to the paper liners. Oops! Yet no matter how messed up your muffins might look, the result will taste good. You could always scrape out the edible parts in a bowl, and pick them up like cookie crumbs. Or if too dry, pour almond milk on top and eat them like cereal. Life—and recipes—are about improvising and going with the flow.

» VEGGIE MILLET HASH BROWNS WITH RADIANCE CARROT KETCHUP (page 217). The recipe is pretty delicious, and that protein-filled millet mashup does resemble potatoes here. Sometimes, though, hash browns can get a little crumbly in the pan . . . or a lot. Maybe they fell apart and become little, mini, baby hash browns in bite-size pieces. It's okay! Scoop them up anyway and eat them. Who says any recipe you make has to look like the picture to taste good?

» DOUBLE CHOCOLATE CHIP AND OATMEAL COOKIES (page 266). As I mention in several places throughout this book, gluten-free, vegan, properly food combined baking is not the easiest thing! Maybe you measured the gluten-free flour mix wrong or packed it in super densely, and your cookies are weird or rock-hard. Hey, they are just cookies after all. Throw them out if you need to, snack on the leftover chocolate chips, and have a good belly laugh.

"That sounds amazing," Melanie said. "I don't know if I can just push my kids out of the bed. I feel bad. . . ."

I replied, "I think it will be better for you *and* for

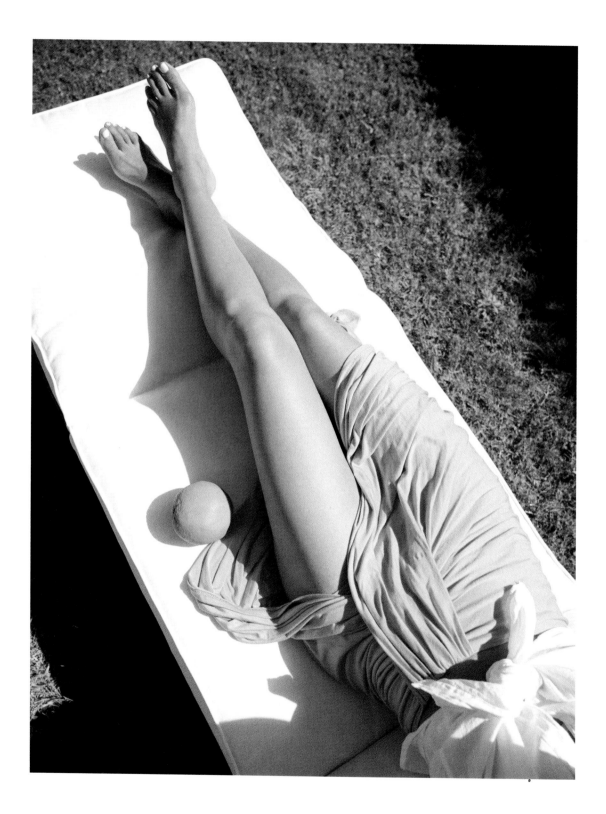

them. And if you work and also do kids' stuff twenty-four hours a day the way you have been, you are going to burn yourself out."

"You're right. I just have to figure out how!"

Melanie never gets anything for herself, and a lot of her activities on the weekends revolve around playdates. With all she has to do, her life is pretty much planned down to every detail. She wasn't prioritizing creating more balance for herself.

Like so many women, Melanie suffers from a guilt complex. Not doing enough at home, not achieving enough, not being good enough, not cooking enough, or whatever. No matter how much gets done, it will never, ever be enough!

Usually, guilt is not truly rooted in reality. We get locked into certain perceptions and think we are "bad" or not good enough or not doing enough, like a hamster on a wheel that never gets anywhere. What guilt is really about is feeling invalid or not fully worthy in some way. We have to keep "doing" more to gain worth, love, or approval. It goes deep. It can stem from a belief we took on in our distant pasts. Henri J. M. Nouwen writes in *The Return of the Prodigal Son* how "they," which he refers to as the voices of society and the outer world, keep us from connecting to our truth:

They suggest that I am not going to be loved without my having earned it through determined efforts and hard work. They want me to prove to myself and others that I am worth being loved, and they keep pushing me to do everything possible to gain acceptance. They deny loudly that love is a totally free gift.

The truth is that we don't have to do anything to be fully worthy. This is part of the never-ending cycle of

life detox recipe

The antidote for guilt is affirming—to ourselves—that we are already worthy just as we are. That's who has to believe it. While it can take some time to truly embody this truth day to day, we can start today to make recipes that say to us, "Yep, you are worth this amazing nourishment!" Here are some great, self-worth-confirming recipes:

» SELF-LOVE CAULIFLOWER SOUP (page 162). Cauliflower is high in vitamins and minerals, and can help balance hormones, reduce inflammation, and improve digestion and detoxification. How's that for self-love?

» NOURISH STEW WITH WHITE BEANS (page 170). This stew not only tastes great—with its Italian herbs and other good things—but it is packed with protein, antioxidants, and minerals. And what I love about stews is that you can't just inhale them; their heat forces you to slow down a bit and give yourself all that amazing nourishment, one spoonful at a time.

» CURRIED RADIANCE CARROT SOUP (page 164). Okay, another soup. I do believe soups and stews, as warming and grounding as they are, are some of the best ways, foodwise, to practice love and care for ourselves! This one comes out a brilliant color from all that wonderful beta-carotene, which converts to vitamin A and helps create healthy skin as it strengthens our immunity.

guilt, as we can never "do" enough if that is where we are trying to get our self-worth. Realizing this is the first step in breaking free of the cycle.

I'm happy to say that Melanie is now in the process of creating a set bedtime for her daughter, Eloise, who has moved into a crib in the nursery. She is working on getting her son to stick to his bedtime, too, so she can have time to herself every evening, free of work and family duties. After I told her about a hiking trip I took to Sedona, she was inspired to plan a trip there and leave the kids with her mom . . . and not feel guilty about it!

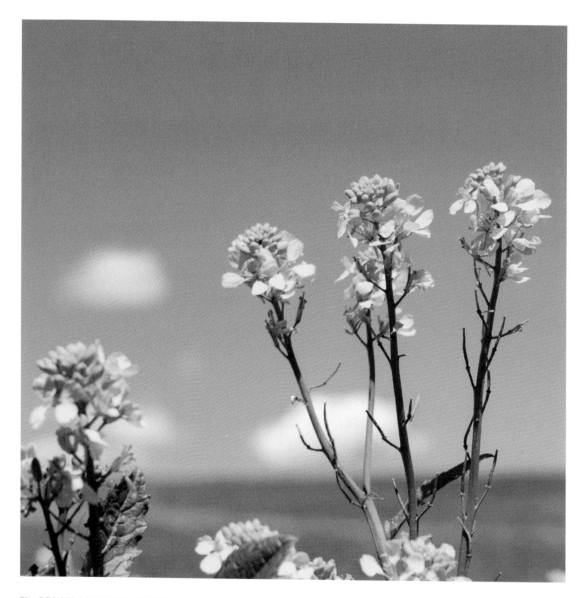

the real source of our worth

If we go within seeking to quiet and ease our minds and thoughts, if we travel to the very deepest core of us, beyond our physical appearance, job title, family life, personality—all of it—we will find a spark. Call it divine light, call it the source of all sources, call it the universe, the name doesn't matter. But this spark connects us to everything else in the world and beyond. We don't earn this spark. We can't buy it or bargain for it. We can't order it and ship it using Amazon Prime, because we already have it. It's ours now and always. And it is the source of all creation.

It took me a long time to connect with my own inner spark. For years I was running around myself, yet no matter how much I accomplished, I still felt I wasn't quite there yet.

One day during deep meditation near a pool of water, I had a revelation of sorts. I realized right then and there that nothing I could do would ever feel like it was enough. I could sell millions of books, help millions more people, and do everything possible for my son and family, and I was still going to feel this vacancy inside me. But here's the crazy part. I also realized that this void inside me never really existed. It was as if a part of me was masquerading as something else. This vacancy was already filled. That there was no emptiness. I was complete because of that spark inside me. I experienced that truth for the very first time, and when I sat up and went back into the world of "doing," everything felt different. It was a huge "aha!" moment. It was like I had been searching for my car keys for years, only to realize they were already in my pocket.

I knew I was seeking something my whole life, as we all are, and even though I had been practicing yoga and meditation for years and written and spoken publicly about self-love, I hadn't really gotten it until that exact moment. This experience occurred during a difficult period I went through some months after my mom had passed, when I was trying to be strong for my dad and Bubs but my whole life felt destabilized. Maybe sometimes we have to hit rock bottom before we break through.

After that encounter with truth, my life was still the same on the outside: running Solluna, podcasting, writing, chasing Bubs in the yard. Yet my whole inner life had shifted. Things don't feel as serious as they used to, and the need for rushing and endless doing is dropping away. I say "dropping" in the present tense, because it is a big unfolding process, and I'm still in process myself. I still falter and get caught up in daily BS—it's like I forget from time to time that the keys to the car are in my pocket—but the veil has been lifted.

You, too, can reconnect with your true worth, which is your power and your true source of validation and love. Our inner spark *is* the perfection within all of us—it's a part of us—and it can never be taken away. It gives us access to perfect love because it is perfect love. It inspires us to be more loving in our lives. Just reading and internalizing this awareness is a step forward. So is meditation, as well as practicing the Stumbling Block Detox (see page 34) and the Letting Go technique (see page 42). All these exercises help us to free ourselves from old, limiting beliefs and emotions that are blocks and distractions. We can really only feel our spark when we are still and calm.

I'm not speaking "in theory." As someone who has been through the fire, so to speak, and made it to the other side, I know it's necessary to keep moving forward. And you keep moving forward by realizing that there is something inside you that can give you energy and direction when you don't think you have any. And remember, there is nothing wrong with doing, nothing wrong with accomplishing grand goals, or even trying to have it all, but no matter what you do or don't do, you are already fully worthy, fully enough, fully beautiful.

To paraphrase Mary Poppins, you are practically perfect in every way.

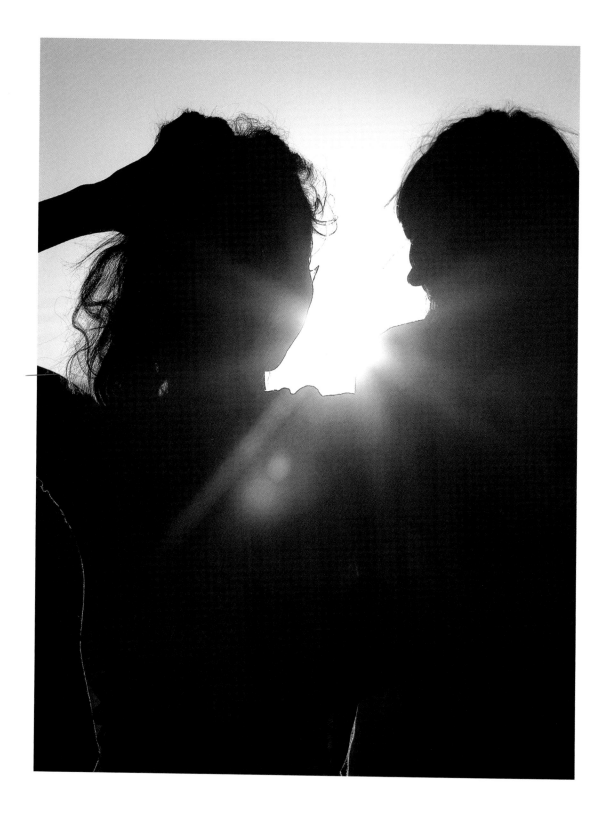

CHAPTER 6

everyone we meet is on a journey, too

Peace, Family, and Food Choices

People are where they are and not where we *want* them to be. No matter how much we wish that our parents or friends ate healthier food or less sugar or processed meat or whatever, they have to make their own decisions. And we need to accept their decisions. It might make us recoil, but pushing others probably makes them want to push back. My dear friend and editor Gary told me that when his friend tells him not to eat hamburgers, it only makes him want to eat them more. The rebelliousness of human nature!

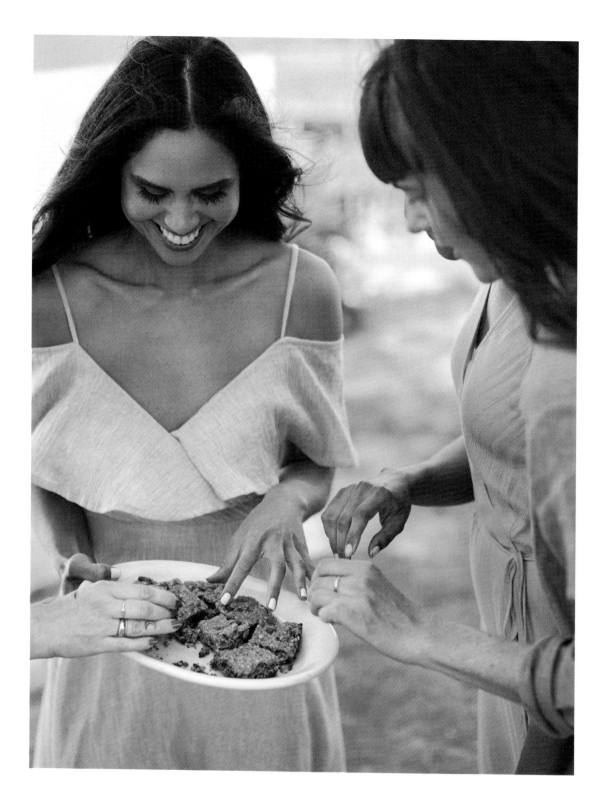

Giving love is more powerful for inspiring change than just throwing more information at someone. We can make large batches of our smoothies and foods, and offer them up for sharing—and be totally okay if this gesture is not accepted. The act of peaceful offering is love itself. Here are some great shareable recipes:

» THE GLOWING GREEN SMOOTHIE (aka GGS; page 99). Yes, it's green, and yes, I know that a lot of people (perhaps including some of your family members!) are scared of all things green! Yet this is *the* recipe that has turned thousands and thousands into GGS lovers, getting their vitamins, minerals, antioxidants, and a boatload more fiber each and every day they drink it. If someone is wanting and willing to drink a few ounces of it, they might just be hooked on the sustained energy they feel and keep going back to the GGS magic. My dad, who did not grow up an ardent vegetable eater, would only drink tiny amounts of the GGS for a few years, then all of a sudden—on his own—he started drinking (and loving!)

big glassfuls, which he now has daily. People need to do things in their own time.

» ALL VEGGIE CLEAN LASAGNA WITH EASY RED SAUCE (page 185). Though it's all veggie, the sauce, plant-based cheese, and organic, non-GMO soy crumbles (if you choose to include them) have a familiar gooey and yummy texture that some loved ones might enjoy. This dish might be a nice intro to nondairy and nonmeat recipe alternatives.

» ENERGIZING PISTACHIO HEMPSEED CUCUMBER SALAD WITH ORANGE ZEST (page 115). This salad is so delicious that non-salad-loving loved ones might just jump on the salad bandwagon . . . at least for this one. They might be shocked at how tasty salad can be without shredded cheese, bottled salad dressings, fried croutons, and so on. It also introduces some interesting ingredients, such as omega-3-rich hempseeds, which might spark some curiosity that expands into new food ingredients. Or not. Either way, it's all good!

As challenging as it can be to witness, we can really only respect others' journey and their choices and allow them their own direct experiences to learn whatever lessons they need to in their time. This includes food and diet. Judging and preaching often get us only to a place of frustration.

I've shared with some relatives the reasons that I encourage eating plant foods and less meat and dairy. They've read parts of my books, and I've typed up a few packets of customized recipes for them. I've cooked for them, emailed them studies and articles. We even watched the provoking documentary *What the Health* together.

Then one night when we were together on a vacation, members of the extended family went out and bought a bunch of blackened, barbecued chicken and gravy.

The charred, carcinogen-filled kind of chicken that was specifically recommended to be avoided on the Harvard Eating Plate (a revision of the government food recommendations by Harvard University), which I had shared with them. *WTF?!* I was dumbfounded. *Did they not understand how bad this is for them? I had told them so!*

I tried to hold it in, but I couldn't help ask, "I'm just curious, for my own work and understanding. . . . How could you see that documentary and know all you know now and still eat the charred meat?" One relative simply said, "I just don't think eating it is that bad."

Wow. Simple as that. It was as clear an answer as I could ever hope or ask for, and it put an abrupt but satisfyingly clear end to the conversation.

I finally got it. No matter how passionately I believe in my dietary philosophy, I can't *make* them or anyone else see it that way. Even if I believe so strongly in my heart that drinking Glowing Green Smoothies and eating veggies is healthy, and that charred, processed meats are not healthy and should be avoided—backing it up with medical studies and nutritional evidence—it wasn't the way it appeared to them.

Everyone has a right to live as they choose. No matter how many food facts or studies we throw at anyone, it may never get them to agree with us. We all simply have different perspectives.

Now I don't feel any pressure to try to persuade these relatives to eat healthier, and I am sure they are also thrilled that I have let it go. I still offer to share healthy dishes I make when we are together, but I've given up pushing. On a more recent visit, they ate a sausage and pepperoni pizza for dinner while I had my veggie bean soup and salad. And we had a really nice conversation about all kinds of topics, none of them nutrition related.

So what's the takeaway from this story? Focus on what's within your power. Don't try to teach by preaching. It rarely works, and often gets you only to a place of frustration. Instead, lead by example. You will exude energy and vitality if you feel good within yourself and about what you are eating, and that is more powerful than anything you can ever say. If anyone asks you about your diet, you can simply tell them that you feel great eating this way, or that it works better for your digestion. Who can argue with that? No need to speak about it further, unless you genuinely think someone would like to know more.

If you live your life in a healthy and faithful way, well, your life is often like a seed that can take root in another's heart. The seed may grow into something extraordinary, and other times it doesn't. Still, be the seed.

Dealing with Bitchiness

When others are mean, downright bitchy, or cutting toward you, remember that their issues are always with themselves. Make a clear separation between their behavior and your feelings about it. Their behavior tells you more about them, and how you react in these situations lets you know more about you.

We're all so focused on our own journeys that we sometimes forget that it's not all about us. Scottish author Ian Maclaren sums it up well with this quote: "Be kind, for everyone you meet is fighting a hard battle." We all deal with crappy negative emotions and struggle to feel balanced and happy at times.

It feels horrible to get the cold shoulder or be treated in a mean or unpleasant way, yet it's a great opportunity to strengthen our compassion muscle. If someone is acting like that, they must surely be in pain and suffering, and they could use some love. Holding the space of love allows you to stay connected to yourself and to them, rather than becoming disconnected *alongside* them.

Some time ago, I gave a talk on wellness and noticed that another wellness speaker I know was in the audience. I couldn't help but be aware of her presence, as well as the fact that her head was buried in her iPhone the whole time. She didn't even look up when I tried to give her a shout-out during my talk! Maybe she was having a bad day. Maybe she was feeling anxious or jealous or some other negative feeling. Maybe she was just plain bored. Who knows? Did I ever learn why she acted this way? No. What I do know is that her behavior didn't have anything to do with me, and there was nothing I could have done to control it or change it. I just gave the best talk I could. So while it admittedly annoyed me a bit, I just shrugged it off. I saw her at an event months later, and I made a point to go up and give her a huge hug

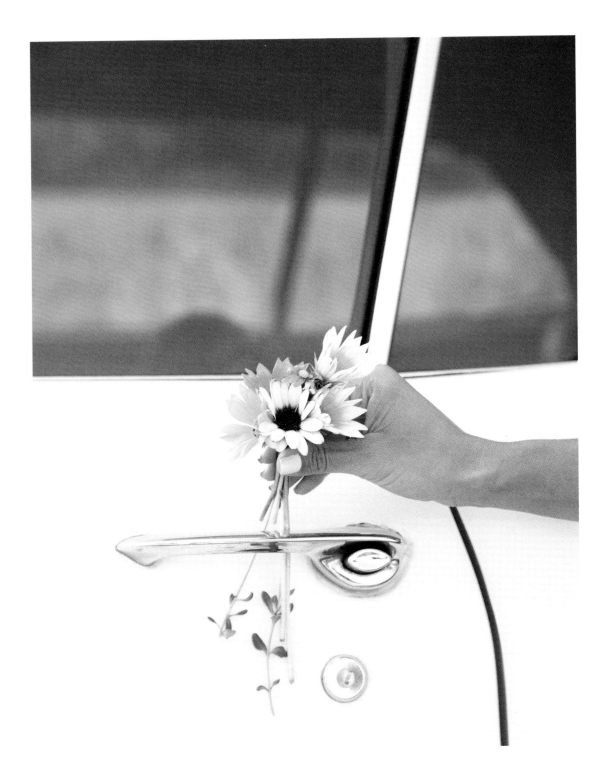

before she could wriggle away. Initially I'm sure she was probably dying to escape, but then I felt her physically start to soften. Love (and hugs!) is the best way to deal with mean, rude, or annoying situations.

Never let others throw you off course, and if they do, don't keep replaying the negativity by telling the story of what happened with so-and-so to your friends over and over again. Take a deep breath and shake it off. Stay connected to your purpose. You can't control others' mood swings or the ways they deal with negative feelings, but you *can* control your own energy and rise above. For a glimpse of what peace doesn't look like, check out some clips of popular, drama-filled reality shows. These give us the gift of inspiring us, shall we say, to go in another direction.

Don't take everyone else's words and expressions so seriously. Your acquaintance's bitchy resting face isn't necessarily there because she thinks you said something stupid, it could be because she is thinking about the fight she just had with her boyfriend. Or maybe your coworker was a bit snappy in her email today because she was upset after just learning that she lost the bid on the house she had her heart set on. Who knows what is flitting through people's minds? We can't. So the only thing to do is to let it all go without overanalyzing.

You can still be strong, and hold healthy boundaries, yet keep them in a loving and compassionate way. We just need to realize that people are where they are on their journeys, and they, too, experience bumps and breakdowns on their imperfect roads of life. Give them space, help when you can, and stay focused on what is kind and beautiful.

life detox recipe

Give yourself supportive foods that can help you feel grounded in the swirl of life and while being around other people's energies. Here are some great recipes for this:

» NATURE'S COMPLETE PROTEIN SMOOTHIE (page 102). This smoothie contains very special fortifying ingredients such as bee pollen and hempseeds. It supplies you with everything from complete proteins, antioxidants, enzymes, and B vitamins to electrolytes, free-radical-scavenging vitamin E, and more. Drink this in the afternoon and have more energy for the rest of your day to stay strong on your life's journey.

» NO-FILTER-NEEDED-SELFIE SMOOTHIE (page 109). You do you, and let your inner glow shine through. You can't worry about what others are thinking. This smoothie is packed with mango for glow-enhancing vitamin C and antioxidants, as well as healthy omega-3 fats from the chia seeds, blood-cleansing turmeric, and digestion-enhancing mint.

» BELLY FEEL GOOD SMOOTHIE (page 110). Sometimes, people's mean comments or actions make your stomach turn. In the process of letting it go (because we know it's better for our health and energy, *not* because what they said or did is okay), we need to be sure to support our gut health. This smoothie contains papaya, which is full of enzymes that support good digestion; ginger, which is also a great digestive; and pineapple, which is full of enzymes including bromelain, which helps to soothe and reduce inflammation and further promotes digestion. Belly feel good indeed!

Closing Thoughts on Life

My views of life, time, and purpose have changed dramatically with the passing of my incredible mother, Sally, on March 29, 2017. She was the one who carried me into life, and her transition rocked my world. Although I know on one level that we are all going to die, she was such a strong force that when she moved on to the next life, it seemed surreal. I curled up next to her in the hospital bed as she slowly took her last breath.

I feel her loving presence even more in my life than when she was in her physical body. Somehow, her passing prompted me to experience an enormous personal expansion, what I can describe as a "cracking open." My heart began to truly unlock for the first time in my life.

Love feels more powerful. More than anything, I now truly realize that ultimately love is the thing that matters most, and the only thing that lasts. I've done intense self-reflection since my mom passed, cleaning up the negative feelings I had inside of me, as well as dispelling the stories and triggers that were present in my life. I made a commitment that going forward I would focus on projecting the most positive energy and supporting everyone I could reach in a deeper way.

While I toyed with the idea of a children's nutrition book and several other projects, the subject matter of this book was the only thing that felt authentic for me to write about at this time.

Beyond the messiness of life, underneath it all, there is perfection. Our true value is not in what we do, but it lies in our being connected to ourselves and others and living from our hearts. No matter what our outer shell (body) looks like, no matter how much or how little money we have, or what we achieve or don't in life, our lovability and validity is always intact. As simple as it sounds, it's a journey to realize this.

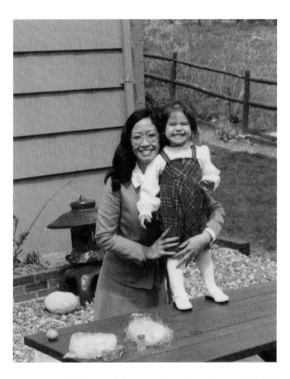

I sincerely hope, with great love, that the offering of this book is of assistance to you on your personal journey. There are no limits to the potential we all have to grow in love, connection, and joy. It's all there already, deep down inside of us, just waiting to awaken.

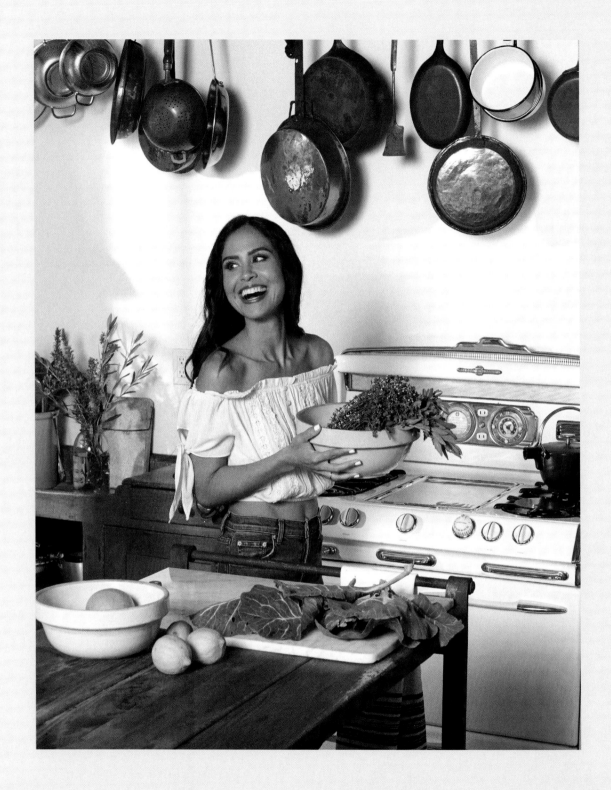

II

Recipes

Now that we've delved into the philosophy behind "perfectly imperfect" in Part I, it's time to dig into some delicious food! Accepting our amazing selves, just as we are, includes detoxing blocks that are physical, emotional, and psychological. How we eat can support healing on all these levels. And all these recipes are designed to be cleansing and rejuvenating in various ways.

Furthermore, all of these recipes are:

» BASED ON WHOLE FOODS. From zucchini to quinoa, working from scratch with a bevy of nutrient-dense whole foods is what these recipes are based in. There are only a few exceptions, such as perfectly imperfect vegan cheese, so you can enjoy these recipes knowing you are supporting your wholeness with whole foods!

» 100 PERCENT PLANT-BASED. Plant foods are the most nutrient-dense, nourishing foods on the planet, and only plant foods contain cleansing fiber! While you don't have to be 100 percent plant-based if you choose not to be at this time, in the spirit of my mantra "Progress, not perfection," the closer to an all plant-based diet you eat, the more cleansed and lighter in your body you will feel, as you gain strength, increased energy, beautiful skin and hair, and more focus.

Besides the astounding nutrition of plant foods, eating plant based is a compassionate, loving way to eat for ourselves and for Mother Nature, our energy (which absorbs and integrates what we eat), and our fellow animals.

» 100 PERCENT GLUTEN-FREE. Gluten can be difficult for many to digest, so all recipes are free of wheat, barley, and rye, as well as products that contain them, like regular soy sauce.

» PROPERLY FOOD COMBINED. Properly combining your foods can lead to more energy; healthier, more glowing skin; an easier time losing weight and slimming down; and more mental clarity. Why? Because digestion is a very energy-intensive process, and if we strategically make digestion easier on our bodies with the combinations of foods we eat at the same time, we can free up large amounts of our own vital energy. For instance, we don't combine dense proteins (like almonds) in a salad with sweet fruit (like blueberries), because the fruit digests much faster than the protein, and it could get stuck in your stomach, creating a traffic jam and the ensuing bloat that follows. For all the information on food combining you could ever want, please check out my first book, *The Beauty Detox Solution*. In the meantime, rest assured that all recipes in this book are properly food combined, so you have nothing to worry about.

Here are some other things I want to highlight in this section:

WHY OUR RECIPES CONTAIN NO GARLIC AND LIMITED ONION

This may come as a surprise to my long-term readers, considering that garlic and onions are cited as some of my top "beauty foods" in my second book, *The Beauty Detox Foods*, and my prior recipes contained these very ingredients so often! To be clear, these foods have definitely been shown to have benefits for our physical health, including garlic's positive effect on cardiovascular health, and the flavonoid antioxidant quercetin and vitamin E found within onions.

I'm constantly learning myself, and the more I go along, the more my work expands beyond just foods and their physical effect on the body to a holistic lifestyle approach that involves our psychological, mental, and spiritual wellness.

In Ayurvedic philosophy, onions and garlic are described as promoting a *rajasic* temperament, which is a hyperactive, restless state. When I studied yoga, I learned that some great yoga masters, including Yogananda, recommended reducing these foods in order to keep the mind calmer for meditation. And when I was traveling in India, I learned that the Jain religion strictly forbids consuming onions or garlic.

I decided to give it a try and have been purposely avoiding garlic and onions in my own diet (except at restaurants, where they sometimes sneak in!) and my recipes. I feel calmer in general myself, and so I keep finding ways to flavor foods without them. There are still onions in some of these recipes, when I felt it really added something, though I totally nixed the garlic. You can try eliminating them yourself and see if you notice a difference in your temperament, increased calmness, and an easier time going deeper in your meditations!

THE IMPORTANCE OF WHOLE GRAINS

It can be confusing when there are conflicting things you hear, such as whole grains are great for you and, on the other hand, you should avoid all grains—even in their whole form! It's literally the opposite advice coming from different factions of experts. In cases like these, it's important to take a step back and look at the bigger picture. First of all, billions around the world live long, healthy lives on a grain-based diet.

In the Okinawa Centenarian Study, researchers found that rice was a dietary staple before Western influence in 1949. After that point, however, when Okinawans began consuming less rice as a proportion of their calories, their health collectively declined and disease became more prevalent. And when a Harvard research team studied more than 110,000 healthy men and women for about twenty-five years, they discovered that those who avoided whole grains in general had an increased risk of heart disease.

I do recommend including gluten-free whole grains, such as quinoa and millet (which are actually both seeds but treated as grains), brown rice, oats, teff, and amaranth as part of a balanced diet. Such grains are a great source of energy, minerals, vitamins, and protein. I also recommend avoiding gluten, which is a protein found in wheat, barley, and rye, as it can be difficult for many to digest and lead to more serious issues in those with celiac disease.

Often, when one tries to avoid grains, they end up going heavy on animal protein. And we know from a great body of research that diets that are high in animal fat and protein correlate strongly with higher rates of disease, including heart disease and cancer of the prostate, breast, and colon. Excessive animal protein puts a heavy burden on digestion, which is energy exhaustive and taxes the liver and kidneys. A study in the journal *Cell Metabolism* found that a person with high animal-protein consumption (meaning over 20 percent of calories come from meat) is four times more likely to die from cancer, a similar rate to that of cigarette smokers.

Ultimately, my goal is not to preach or "win" any kind of argument or debate with proponents of higher animal-food-based diets. Each of us must listen to our own bodies and hearts and what we feel is true and best. My intention for this discussion is simply to offer how I feel—that a whole food, plant-based diet including vegetables, fruit, nuts, seeds, legumes, and gluten-free grains is a beautiful and powerfully rejuvenating way to support our highest health and vitality.

ORGANIC SOY IS OKAY IN MODERATION

Soybeans have been consumed by humans for thousands of years. They originated in Southeast Asia and were first domesticated by Chinese farmers about 1100 BC. They started to be grown in Japan and other countries by the first century AD and have been a mainstay in many Asian cultures since then.

Soybeans are a rich source of protein, yielding more protein per acre of land than any other crop. Soybeans are also high in minerals like iron, manganese, phosphorus, copper, potassium, magnesium, zinc, selenium, and calcium. They are abundant in essential vitamins, including riboflavin, folate, vitamin B_6, vitamin K, thiamin, and vitamin C. Even among plant foods, soybeans are one of the highest sources of fiber available.

When we consume soy, it absolutely must be organic and non-GMO to prevent further contamination of our food supply by genetically modified organisms. Whole soy foods are the kinds we can consume (as long as you don't have a soy allergy, of course), which are minimally processed, so they retain the most nutritional benefits. Whole soy options include tofu and edamame, as well as tempeh, miso, and natto, made of fermented cooked soybeans. Tamari, a gluten-free soy sauce which is the liquid by-product that forms when making miso paste, is also okay to consume. What we must avoid are highly processed soy products, such as the ones included in junk food, like soy protein isolates, soybean oil, and so on.

In *The Beauty Detox Solution*, I recommended consuming tempeh and miso in moderation. So what changed from my first book to now, and why am I okay with consuming more tofu, which is not a processed form of soy, yet still not one of my original fermented forms? Because of newer research and investigating the validity of the anti-soy information.

Soy has been accused of containing estrogen. It doesn't; soy contains phytoestrogens, which are healthy compounds found in other antioxidant-rich plant foods. (Dairy milk does contain real estrogen, however.)

Another popular myth is that soy negatively alters sex hormones in men, contributing to the dreaded "man boobs." However, in several studies examining soy protein or isoflavone supplementation, there were no significant changes in testosterone, free testosterone, estrogen, sex-hormone-binding globulin protein, or semen quality of the men studied.

Okay, okay—but what about soy's negative effects on thyroid or, worse, cancer? In one extensive research summary published in the journal *Thyroid* that analyzed the results of fourteen clinical trials, it was concluded that in healthy, iodine-replete individuals, neither soy foods nor isoflavones adversely affect thyroid function.

There has been back and forth on the connection between soy and breast cancer, but a recent, sizable study involving over 6,200 women with breast cancer between 1995 and 2015 has "put that argument to rest," according to Dr. Omer Kucuk, a medical oncologist at Emory University's Winship Cancer Institute, who has studied soy isoflavones. In fact, the 2017 study, published in the journal *Cancer*, found that soy was actually associated with a decreased risk of death related to breast cancer.

There are two to three daily servings of soy in the traditional Japanese diet, delivering 25 to 50 milligrams of isoflavones (phytoestrogens) per day, which appears to have protective benefits, according to research published in the *American Journal of Clinical Nutrition*.

Overall, an entire book could be written dispelling the many myths about soy. Of course, that doesn't mean I'm not concerned about GMO soy (which is rampant and should be avoided), or highly processed soy foods (also popular and to be avoided). My position is now simply that some organic, whole, soy-based foods can be a part of a healthy diet.

CHOOSE ORGANIC WHENEVER POSSIBLE!

Choosing organic is superimportant for our true health, as well as the entire planet. In order to be our most healthy, radiant, beautiful, and energetic selves, we need to avoid exposure to toxic chemicals. Nonorganic agriculture uses billions of pounds of chemical pesticides and herbicides annually.

Besides, organically grown foods are more flavorful and contain more nutrients, including more vitamins, minerals, enzymes, and micronutrients, than commercially grown foods. The *Journal of Alternative and Complementary Medicine* conducted a review of forty-one published studies comparing the nutritional value of organically grown and conventionally grown fruits, vegetables, and grains, and concluded that there are significantly more of certain nutrients, including iron, vitamin C, phosphorus, and magnesium, in organic foods crops.

Organic foods also cannot be tampered with for genetic engineering (GE) or made into GMO foods, of which we fully understand the detrimental and long-term repercussions.

Choosing organic is also the best thing to do to support farming that is in harmony with nature, which includes crop rotation for healthier soil, more biodiversity, and better support for the larger ecosystem. It helps to reduce pollution and protects our water and soil from agricultural chemicals, pesticides, and fertilizers that contaminate our environment and all the other species that also call Earth their home as well.

If budget is an option, please consult the Environmental Working Group's (www.ewg.org) list of the Dirty Dozen and the Clean Fifteen for guidance on the most important foods to put your dollars toward.

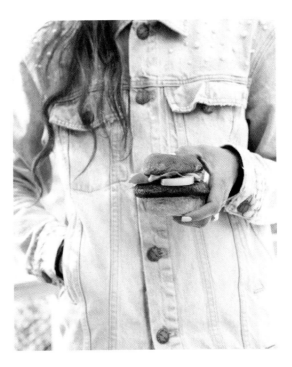

FREQUENTLY USED INGREDIENTS AND WHERE TO FIND THEM

Some ingredients used in our recipes might be less familiar. I want to be sure to highlight them in this section so you can start feeling comfortable (i.e., become friends!) with them. I include some information on why they are special and tips on where to find them for your own kitchen.

ACAI. Acai berries are superhigh in antioxidants, vitamin C, detoxifying fiber, and minerals such as potassium and calcium, and are naturally sugar-free. Acai can be purchased in smoothie packets in the frozen-fruit section. My favorite brand, which I've been using for years, is the Sambazon unsweetened variety.

ALMOND BUTTER. Almonds are an excellent beauty food, full of minerals, antioxidants, vitamin E, and protein. You can find almond butter in the nut-butter section of markets, or even made fresh at your local supermarket!

ALMOND FLOUR. This gluten-free flour is high in fiber and protein, which benefits digestion and healthy weight loss. It also promotes heart health and energy levels, and can be found in the baking section with other flours or online.

ALMOND MILK. A great source of calcium and vitamin E. Made from blending the mighty almond with water and then squeezing out the pulp, it reduces blood pressure, strengthens muscles, and improves kidney health. It is easy to prepare yourself (see page 100) or to source at a grocery store in the milks section.

ALOE JUICE. Sourced from the superresilient, beautiful aloe plant, this juice is extremely hydrating and highly alkaline. It improves liver function and aids in ridding the body of toxic waste. It also contains enzymes that help break down fats and sugars to improve digestion. Aloe juice can be found at a health market or online.

ANISEEDS. These seeds are similar in flavor to licorice root and regulate blood sugar, block the growth of fungus and bacteria, and have been used medicinally to aid in digestive and hormonal problems. Aniseeds can be found in the spice section of markets or online.

ARROWROOT POWDER. This root starch acts as a thickener and is an important ingredient in gluten-free baking recipes. It has been known to boost immune function and fight foodborne allergens. You can find this in the baking section of your local health food store or online.

ASHWAGANDHA. This is a powerful rejuvenating herb that has the ability to relieve stress and protect brain cells against the effects of our fast-paced lifestyle. What's even more special about ashwagandha is that it does not act as a stimulant. This herb can most easily be sourced at health food markets or online. Along with other herbs, it's important to source only organic.

BEE POLLEN. Bee pollen is approximately 25 percent complete bioavailable protein (50 percent more protein by weight than beef). In addition, bee pollen provides more than a dozen vitamins, including B vitamins, twenty-eight minerals, enzymes or coenzymes, beneficial fatty acids, and antioxidants. The best place to get bee pollen is from a local, ethical beekeeper who treats his or her bees with love and care!

BLACK PEPPER. See Freshly ground black pepper (versus preground).

BROWN RICE FLOUR. This flour is a nutritious, naturally gluten-free alternative to white flour. It is rich in iron, fiber, vitamin B, manganese, and protein. If you have not yet tried brown rice flour, you will find it has a fuller, nuttier flavor than wheat flour. It can be found at your local health food store in the baking section.

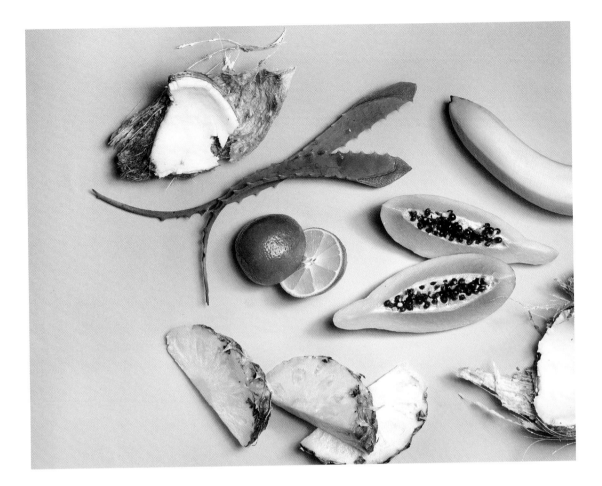

CACAO. Cacao is the raw form of the cacao bean, which is less processed—and has powerful antioxidant effects and health benefits. Cacao also contains anandamide, a neurotransmitter called the "bliss molecule." You may choose to purchase cacao at any health food store or online. Be sure to source organic!

CARDAMOM. This spice is excellent for muscle and joint pain and gastrointestinal disorders. The oils and biochemicals in cardamom are also extremely detoxifying. You can find pods as well as ground cardamom in the spice section. For our recipes here, we are using ground.

CASHEWS. Cashews are a healthy source of dietary fat, which means they promote heart health and lower bad cholesterol. They are also high in magnesium, which aids in the development of muscles, bones, and organs. You can find them in the nuts and seeds section of markets.

CHIA SEEDS. Chia seeds an incredible, clean source of omega-3 fatty acids. They have excellent cleansing and detoxifying properties, as well as the ability to help maintain blood sugar levels and aid in weight loss. They also offer protein, antioxidants, vitamins, and a variety of minerals, like calcium. You can find chia seeds at many markets today in the nuts and seeds section or online.

CINNAMON. Cinnamon is a potent rejuvenating spice that can boost metabolism, help stabilize blood sugar, cure sugar cravings between meals, and control blood sugar levels. It is full of antioxidants that protect the body from oxidative damage and reduce inflammation. You can find cinnamon in the spice section.

COCONUT FLAKES. Coconut flakes are a great topping that create a crunchy texture and contain a small amount of phosphorus, iron, carbs, and protein. You can source them in the baking section of markets or online. Look for unsweetened varieties.

COCONUT MILK. This rich, fatty plant milk derives from the amazing coconut. It contains beneficial fatty acids such as lauric acid, which help increase energy levels and lower blood pressure. Its medium-chain triglycerides help provide energy and burn fat. You can find coconut milk in the milks section, in the aisle with other cartons of plant milks, or in the Asian section of grocery stores.

COCONUT NECTAR. This sweet syrup contains up to seventeen amino acids, an abundance of minerals, and vitamins B and C. It is also low on the glycemic index and very low in fructose in comparison to other liquid sweeteners (such as agave). You can find coconut nectar in the grocery store (look in the aisle with other syrups and honey) or online.

COCONUT OIL. This oil is excellent for high-heat cooking as it has a higher smoke point, meaning it retains its integrity at higher temperatures, and won't break down and create free radicals. It can even boost digestion and energy as it contains short- and medium-chain fatty acids. You can find it at the grocery store next to other cooking oils. Look for unrefined, virgin, organic varieties.

COCONUT SUGAR. This is a great alternative to white granulated sugar because it is much lower on the glycemic index. It is packed with vitamins, minerals, and phytonutrients and can be found at your local health food store next to the other sugars.

COCONUT YOGURT. This dairy-free alternative is packed with probiotics (though, as with all yogurts, it does not replace an excellent probiotics supplement) and is a great source of bone-building calcium. You can find it in the refrigerated yogurt section.

CORIANDER. The essential oils of borneol and linalool in coriander help to promote digestion and proper liver function. Ayurveda also believes it is beneficial in creating beautiful skin and healthy hair. You can find ground coriander in the spice section of the market.

CRANBERRIES. Cranberries act as a natural diuretic by stimulating your kidneys to flush excessive fluids out of your body, thereby helping to prevent bloating and excess water weight. This berry is also full of antioxidants. For the two ways cranberries are used in these recipes, you can source them dried in the dried fruit aisle or bulk bins, and also frozen in the frozen fruit section.

CUMIN. According to Ayurveda, cumin is an excellent spice for improving digestion and eliminating toxins.

You can find ground cumin in the spice section. Whole cumin seeds can also be sourced in the spice aisle, though they are a bit more rare, and can also be found online.

DATES. Medjool dates are a great source of fiber, calcium, and are also rich in copper, an important mineral that the body uses to help absorb iron, form collagen and red blood cells, create a healthy nervous system, and generate energy. Dates can be found in the dried-fruit aisle of markets or, sometimes, in the produce section.

FIGS. The tiny seeds of figs are packed with nutrients that help cleanse the digestive tract of toxins and mucus. Excess mucus in the digestive tract prevents your body from absorbing vital nutrients, so integrating figs is a must! Figs can be found in the dried-fruit section of markets or online.

FLAX OIL. This oil is packed with healthy omega-3s and fatty acids that promote heart health, improve mood, and decrease inflammation. Flax oil can quickly oxidize and needs to be refrigerated. You can find it at your local health food store in the refrigerated section.

FRESHLY GROUND BLACK PEPPER. Freshly ground black pepper aids in healthy digestion because it increases the hydrochloric acid in the stomach. It is preferable to get a pepper grinder and grind your peppercorns fresh into recipes for more flavor, and to prevent the natural oils from going rancid. Check out pepper grinders and peppercorns at home-goods stores and groceries.

GARBANZO BEAN FLOUR (AKA CHICKPEA FLOUR). This excellent gluten-free flour is made from ground chickpeas and is high in protein, fiber, and iron. It acts as an excellent binder in recipes, eliminating the need for processed egg replacers. It's inexpensive and essential to make all these delicious Perfectly Imperfect recipes! Look for garbanzo bean flour in the baking section of markets; if you have trouble sourcing it locally, you can always order it online.

GOJI BERRIES. This renowned berry is packed with antioxidants, B vitamins, and polysaccharides, has eighteen kinds of amino acids, and is a rich source of potassium and fiber. The berries contain adaptogens that increase our resistance to stress, anxiety, and fatigue. You can find goji berries at your local health food store or in Asian markets. It's fun to go to Chinatown to find goji berries!

GUAR GUM. This gluten-free and vegan powder is made from guar beans and is used for thickening and stabilizing ingredients in gluten-free baking. It is also low in calories and high in fiber. It is a great alternative to other emulsifying agents such as carrageenan. You can find this ingredient in the baking section of a health food store.

HEMP MILK. Hemp milk is made from the seeds of the hemp plant and is a fantastic plant-based milk to rotate in. Hemp contains skin-, heart-, and brain-supporting omega-3 fatty acids, protein, vitamins, and minerals such as zinc. You can find it in the milks section of the market, or try making your own (see page 101).

HEMPSEEDS. Hempseeds are an incredible rejuvenation food. They are a perfect blend of easily digested

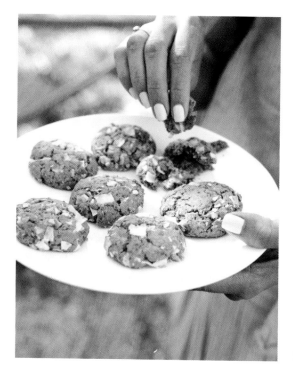

which is key for cleansing the liver, our main detoxifying organ. You can find lemons at the grocery store or, depending where you live, at your local farmers' market.

MAPLE SYRUP. This syrup contains polyphenol antioxidants and adds a rich, sweet taste. It is lower on the glycemic index than white granulated sugar or agave. You can find this syrup in the aisle with the sweeteners. Be sure to source pure maple syrup over ones mixed with inferior sweeteners like high-fructose corn syrup!

MILLET. This incredibly nutritious, fortifying grain is technically a seed. It contains a great deal of amino acids to build protein in the body. It also contains the important nutrients of manganese, magnesium, calcium, zinc, iron, B vitamins, vitamins E and K, and fiber. You can find millet in the bulk section with the grains, or in bags in the grain and beans aisle.

protein, essential omega-3 fats, gamma linolenic acid (GLA), antioxidants, fiber, iron, calcium, zinc, carotene, and vitamins. Hempseeds are usually found in the nuts and seeds section at the market or sometimes in the supplement section, or they can be sourced online.

KELP NOODLES. This sea-vegetable-based noodle is virtually calorie-free and is an amazing all-veggie noodle replacement. It contains vitamins A and C, as well as the B vitamins and minerals like magnesium, calcium, zinc, and iron. Kelp noodles are found suspended in water in little bags in the refrigerated section of health food markets, or look online.

LEMONS. Lemons are one of the most detoxifying foods around. They contain vitamin C and enzymes that boost the liver's function and tissue regeneration,

MISO PASTE. Miso is a nutritious, rejuvenating food that contains probiotics and antioxidants that promote immunity and balance gut bacteria. The two forms we use in these recipes are white miso, which is made from soybeans that have been fermented along with rice, and red miso, which has a longer fermentation period. Miso can be found in the refrigerated section of health food stores and at Asian markets.

NORI SEAWEED. Nori is a type of seaweed that is made into high-mineral, virtually calorie-free sheets that can be used to roll sushi or as the base for simple little wraps (like the Ananda Burrito in *The Beauty Detox Solution*). It is packed with B vitamins and iodine, calcium, and iron. Nori can be found in the Asian section at health food stores or online.

NUTRITIONAL YEAST. These yellow flakes boast an extremely rich source of easily assimilated amino acids to create protein in your body, over fourteen key minerals, and seventeen vitamins, including the B vitamins. It is often fortified with B_{12}, which helps to create strong hair, nails, and skin, and fight fatigue. You can find nutritional yeast in the bins or supplement aisle at your local health food store or online.

OATS. See Quick-cooking oats; Steel-cut oats.

ORGANIC SOY CRUMBLES. Organic soy crumbles are great for transitioning the diet from animal protein to plant protein as they have a hearty texture and are high in protein. Be sure to source all of your soy products as organic and non-GMO. You can find soy crumbles alongside tofu in the refrigerated section of the market, which is sometimes labeled the "Meat Alternatives" section.

PUMPKIN SEEDS. These seeds are an excellent source of zinc, sulfur, and vitamin A. They are also a rich source of essential fatty acids and cell-protecting vitamins C, E, and K. Pumpkin seeds supply a good amount of protein, along with magnesium, calcium, phosphorus, manganese, copper, and iron. You can find them in the nuts and seeds section.

QUICK-COOKING OATS. These are an excellent source of a powerful fiber called beta-glucan, which helps reduce blood sugar and cholesterol levels. Oats are packed with minerals and vitamins such as zinc, iron, and folate! While long-cooking steel-cut oats are a great complex, energizing fuel source, quick-cooking oats are perfect for a crunchier texture in certain recipes, such as our Wholesome Banana Crisp (page 250). You can find quick-cooking oats in the bulk section or in the cereal aisle.

QUINOA. Quinoa is strengthening without being heavy or dense. It is a great source of protein and contains all nine essential amino acids. It also happens to be gluten-free, anti-inflammatory, and high in minerals. This grain-like seed can be found in the bulk section or in the aisle with the rice and pasta.

RAW APPLE CIDER VINEGAR (ACV). This is a liver and lymphatic tonic that can help detox your body. It not only helps to balance your body's pH, but it also supports elimination, lymphatic drainage, and lower blood sugar levels. The best apple cider vinegar should be made from certified organic apples and sourced raw. It can easily be found at health food stores in the oil and vinegar section.

SEA SALT. Sea salt is minimally processed, so its abundance of dozens of trace minerals remains intact and it is preferable over denatured table salt. Look for sea salt in the spice section.

SESAME OIL. In Ayurvedic philosophy, sesame seed oil is considered one of the most powerfully warming oils, helping to boost circulation and metabolism. However, sesame seed oil is a rich, concentrated source of omega-6 fats, which most of us get too much of, so we use this oil sparingly. Look for sesame oil alongside other oils or in the Asian section at grocery stores.

SESAME SEEDS. These tiny seeds are amazing storehouses of antioxidants, as well as a rich source of vitamins and minerals, including zinc, magnesium, phosphorus, iron, calcium, and vitamins B and E. Sesame seeds can be sourced in the nuts and seeds section of markets or online.

SORGHUM FLOUR. This flour originated in Africa thousands of years ago, and sorghum is the fifth most important cereal crop in the world. Sorghum flour, an important component of the KS Gluten-Free Flour Mix (page 252), is gluten-free, non-GMO, and low on the glycemic index, which makes it easily digestible and helps balance blood sugar and fight inflammation. It contains protein, iron, fiber, and antioxidants, and creates slower, more sustained energy burn-off. Look for it in the baking section of markets, where gluten-free products are becoming more prevalent, or online.

SPIRULINA. Spirulina is a powerful rejuvenating food that helps us restore our hair and skin health, improves brain function, and boosts immunity and overall health. Spirulina is one of the most complete food sources in the world, with over one hundred nutrients and greater than 60 percent protein content. You can source spirulina online or in the supplement or superfoods section of a health food store.

STEEL-CUT OATS. Steel-cut oats are minimally processed, being cut a few times but not precooked. As such, they tend to retain a higher amount of protein and fiber, and provide long-burning energy. They supply 7 grams of protein per ¼ cup serving, as well as fiber, iron, and B vitamins. Steel-cut oats can be found in grocery stores in the cereal aisle or in the bulk section.

SUNFLOWER SEEDS. These seeds are high in vitamin E, which rids the body of free radicals that cause

cellular damage. They also contain selenium, which promotes DNA repair. You can source sunflower seeds in the nuts and seeds section or in the bulk section.

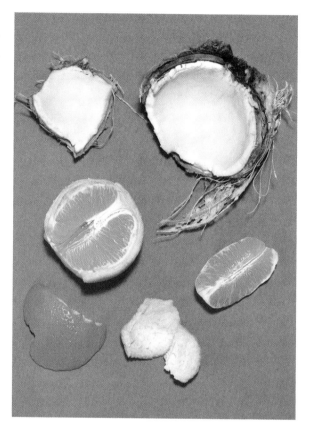

TAHINI. Tahini is made from sesame seeds, which provide both healthy fats and essential amino acids—the building blocks of protein. Tahini also provides vitamin E, B vitamins, trace minerals, and fatty acids. You will also receive your daily copper—needed to maintain nerve, bone, and metabolic health. Look for tahini in the nut-butter section of the market.

TAMARI. This is a gluten-free premium soy sauce that has more nutrients and protein because of the way it is fermented. You can find it at Asian markets, as well as next to the traditional soy sauces at the grocery store.

TAPIOCA FLOUR. This flour helps boost energy levels and is high in iron, which increases circulation. It is a great source of gluten-free fiber, which also promotes healthy digestion. It can be found at your local health food store in the baking section or, if you have any trouble finding it there, online.

TEFF FLOUR. Teff is a wonderful gluten-free grain that is fortifying and contains a good deal of protein. It also contains fiber and minerals such as iron, calcium, and manganese. It is an important ingredient in our KS Gluten-Free Flour Mix (page 252), and is also used to make gluten-free wraps. You can find this in the baking section at your local health food store or online.

TEMPEH, NON-GMO ORGANIC. Tempeh is a vitality-supporting fermented form of soy that is superhigh in protein and more easily digested and assimilated. It can be found in the refrigerated section of markets, next to tofu and sometimes meat, or sometimes in a section labeled "Meat Alternatives."

TOFU, NON-GMO ORGANIC. Tofu is an excellent source of plant-based protein, containing all nine essential amino acids as well as various minerals. For more information on organic soy, see page 85. You can find tofu in the refrigerated section. It is essential to purchase *only* tofu that is labeled non-GMO and organic.

TURMERIC. This powerful fortifying spice is anti-inflammatory, due to a compound it contains called curcumin. It helps to protect our cellular integrity, cleanse the blood, and create healthy blood flow, which in turn gives us glowing skin. You can find ground turmeric, which is what is called for in these recipes, in the spice section of the market.

VANILLA EXTRACT. Vanilla extract is sourced from vanilla beans, which are grown in a vine-like plant that climbs up trees. It contains antioxidants that protect the body and reduce inflammation. You can find vanilla extract in the baking section.

VEGAN CHEESE. Vegan cheese can be made from pea protein, soy, nuts, seeds, vegetable oils, nutritional yeast, or flours. While it is processed and is not a whole food, it is still an excellent transition food that can be enjoyed occasionally as a dairy replacement. Brands such as Daiya or Follow Your Heart are becoming more available in the dairy section of the grocery store.

VEGAN PROTEIN POWDER. Vegan protein powder is a superior option over other varieties, as it is easy to digest and assimilate. I personally recommend only high-quality non-GMO, organic, plant-based options. Look for vegan or plant-based protein powders in the supplement section of health food stores and also online.

YOUNG COCONUT. Some key nutrients contained in coconut are lauric acid, iron, potassium, magnesium, and calcium. Potassium is an electrolyte that helps to facilitate cellular cleansing and is about twice as concentrated in coconut water as in a banana. You can buy young coconuts, which contain their natural meat and water, in the produce section of health food stores or in Asian markets.

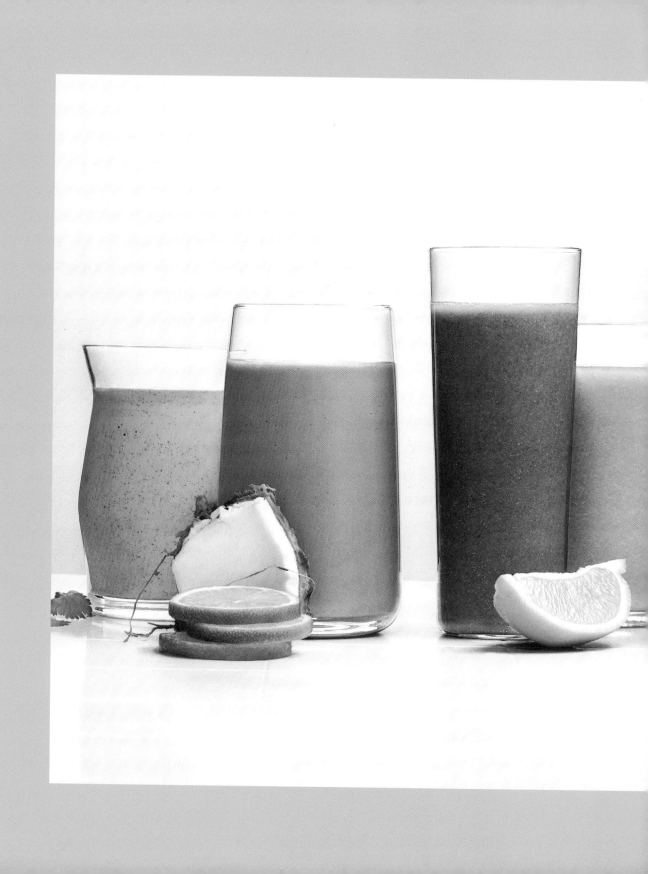

smoothies and bowls

Smoothies are an effective and powerful tool to nourish us. Smoothies respect Mother Nature's inherent wisdom in her whole food creations, for the entire fruit, veggies, seeds, nuts, and so on are blended together, fiber and juice intact.

Smoothies are an important part of our long-term lifestyle; the Glowing Green Smoothie is a key element of our morning practice, but it, as well as these other recipes, can be enjoyed midmorning or midafternoon. If you want even more smoothie options beyond the ones found here, I have tons more recipes to offer on my website, mysolluna.com.

Because they are blended, smoothies are in essence "predigested," meaning we can more easily assimilate their nutrition, while the fiber they contain helps to cleanse our systems and maintain healthy blood sugar and energy levels. Incorporating the ritual of smoothies into your life is an exciting way to say to yourself, "Yes, I am worthy of amazing nourishment!"

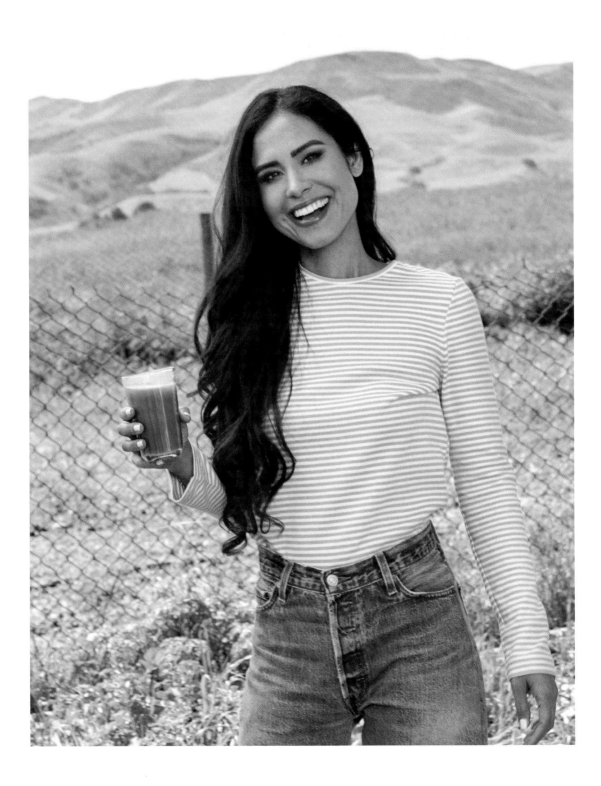

the glowing green smoothie (aka ggs)

**MAKES ABOUT
60 OUNCES, OR
2½ TO 4 SERVINGS**

Here it is . . . the one and only GGS! Packed with everything from radiance-inducing vitamins, enzymes, and minerals to amino acids, antioxidants, and more, this incredible elixir has been featured everywhere from *Good Morning America* to *Vogue*. I do encourage mixing and matching your greens and fruit, but there is a basic ratio to the GGS: around 70 percent dark leafy greens, around 30 percent high-fiber whole fruit, and always the vitamin-C-filled and liver-supporting fresh lemon juice. I encourage keeping it simple and limited to these elements, without adding any concentrated protein (like protein powder) or fat (like chia seeds). Save all those great ingredients for a bit later in the day, and allow the GGS to do its cleansing magic with vitamin-filled fruit as you rebuild with the mineral-rich greens!

As it cleanses and detoxifies your system, the GGS will give you sustained energy; beautiful, glowing skin; true beauty from the inside out; and optimal digestion. It also fosters a focused, clear mind. The GGS is here to support us daily on our life's journey of growth, and it's an integral part of my morning practice.

2 cups cold filtered
    water

1 bunch spinach

3 or 4 celery stalks,
    halved

1 head romaine lettuce

Small bunch cilantro,
    thick stems cut off
    (optional)

Small bunch parsley,
    thick stems cut off
    (optional)

1 apple, cored, seeded,
    and quartered

1 pear, cored, seeded,
    and quartered

1 banana

½ fresh lemon, peeled
    and seeded

Place the water, spinach, celery, romaine, and herbs, if using, into a Vitamix or other blender in the order listed, and secure the lid. Start the blender on low speed, then gradually increase the speed and blend until smooth. Add the apple, pear, banana, and lemon and blend until smooth.

fresh almond milk

Fresh almond milk is delicious and bursting with fresh vitamins and enzymes. An advantage of making your own almond milk is that you can soak and sprout your almonds, which helps to remove the natural phytic acid on the outside of the almonds, thereby increasing the nutrient absorption. It is a great self-love practice to create your own nut milk, pressed fresh in your own kitchen!

1 cup raw unsalted almonds, soaked overnight, rinsed well, and drained

3 cups filtered water

Pinch of sea salt

1. Combine the almonds, water, and sea salt in a blender or food processor. Blend on high speed for about 2 minutes in a blender; if you are using a food processor, you probably need to process for about 4 minutes to get the almonds broken down into a fine enough meal.

2. Strain the almonds by pouring the almond-water mixture through a nut-milk bag or cheesecloth into a bowl, pitcher, or large glass measuring container. Be sure to squeeze the bag or cloth very tightly, obtaining as much almond milk as possible.

3. Store the almond milk in sealed containers in the fridge for up to 2 days.

fresh hemp milk

MAKES ABOUT 4 CUPS

Hempseed, full of essential omega-3 fats, minerals, and protein, is an amazing rejuvenating food to support our muscles, hair, brain power, beautiful skin, hormonal balance, and more. Straining is not necessary, which means it's even easier to make than almond milk. Making hemp milk fresh makes it taste truly alive. Try it for yourself!

½ cup hempseeds

4 cups filtered water (use less water to create a thicker, creamier milk)

Pinch of sea salt

1. Combine the hempseeds, water, and sea salt in a blender, and blend on high speed for about 1 minute, or until the mixture is well combined.

2. Transfer the milk to sealed containers and refrigerate. It will keep in the refrigerator for up to 5 days (note that it stores longer than almond milk—yessss!).

nature's complete protein smoothie

SERVES 1

The power-packed ingredients in this smoothie provide B vitamins, omega-3 fats, complete protein, vitamin E, calcium, antioxidants, and more. Try this recipe when you are looking for an energy boost or as a great post-workout or post-hike option.

1¼ cups Fresh Hemp Milk (page 101), Fresh Almond Milk (page 100), or store-bought hemp or almond milk

2 teaspoons bee pollen

1 tablespoon almond butter

1 tablespoon hempseeds

½ large frozen ripe banana

1 tablespoon coconut nectar

1 teaspoon vanilla extract

Pinch of sea salt

In a blender, combine all the ingredients. Starting on low speed and increasing to high, blend the ingredients together until smooth, about 30 to 45 seconds.

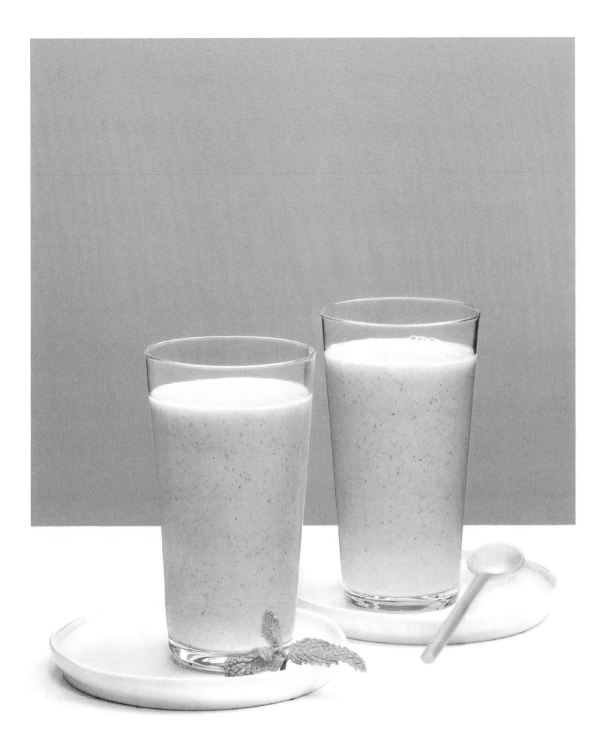

chia gel

**SERVES 3 TO 6
(DEPENDING ON USE)**

Chia seeds are extremely hydrophilic, meaning that they love and are attracted to water. The outside of chia seeds are covered in tiny microfibers, and when soaked in a liquid medium, they can absorb and hold around twelve times their weight in water. This creates a gel of soluble and insoluble fiber that is cleansing and also hydrating.

Spoon this chia gel into smoothie recipes instead of dry chia seeds (as dry chia seeds love water so much they might actually be dehydrating, by absorbing water from our GI tracts). Chia gel can be used as an egg replacer in certain recipes, such as the Superhero Spinach Balls (page 235).

Depending on how much you use chia seeds or how big your household is, you can multiply this recipe to make larger amounts at once. It will keep, stored and covered in the fridge, for up to five days.

⅓ cup chia seeds

2 cups filtered water

In a bowl, combine and stir the chia seeds and filtered water. Cover and let sit for at least 20 minutes, until the chia seeds and water mix evenly and form a thick gel. Stir until thoroughly mixed. Stir again right before serving.

i want it all smoothie

SERVES 1

Ever sit there wondering if your body wants a green smoothie or a protein smoothie? Here you can have both at the same time! This is a green smoothie combined with some hearty, protein-filled almond butter and chia seeds. You'll get it all: protein, minerals, antioxidants, and vitamins. We include only slower-digesting banana, however, for the fruit component, which allows this smoothie to remain properly food combined. This is a great midafternoon boost to propel you to have an amazing, inspiring second half of your day!

1 cup Fresh Almond Milk (page 100) or store-bought unsweetened almond milk

1 cup fresh spinach

1 tablespoon almond butter

2 pitted Medjool dates

2 tablespoons Chia Gel (opposite)

1 medium frozen banana

In a blender, combine all the ingredients. Starting on low speed and then increasing to high, blend until smooth.

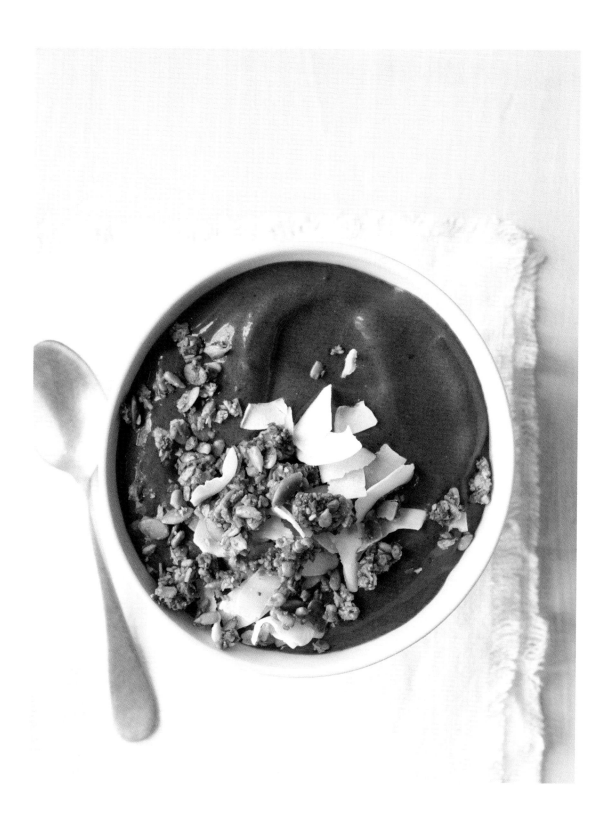

power protein bowl

SERVES 1

Depending on the protein powder you use, this super-nutrient-filled bowl will supply you with upward of 20-plus grams of protein, omega-3 fats, vitamin C, antioxidants, and loads of energy. It's excellent post-workout as a replenishing tonic in a bowl. And sometimes, we might be in the mood to eat a bowl with a spoon, which feels like a little meal, over drinking it in a smoothie!

½ cup Fresh Almond Milk (page 100) or store-bought unsweetened almond milk

2 (100-gram) packets frozen acai (see page 87)

1 serving vegan protein powder (follow suggested serving size)

1½ tablespoons Chia Gel (page 104)

1 tablespoon cacao powder

1 pitted Medjool date

1 teaspoon ashwagandha powder

1 medium frozen banana

Dash of ground cinnamon

Dash of vanilla extract

⅓ cup gluten-free, nut-based granola, for topping

1 tablespoon coconut flakes, for topping

1. In a blender, combine the almond milk, acai, vegan protein powder, Chia Gel, cacao powder, date, ashwagandha, banana, cinnamon, and vanilla extract. Starting on low speed and increasing to high, blend the ingredients together until smooth, about 1 minute.

2. Use a spatula to scrape the mixture into a bowl. Top with the granola and coconut flakes, and enjoy immediately.

happy bunny smoothie

SERVES 2

This beautiful and delicious smoothie is a great boost for healthy skin. It's packed with beta-carotene, which converts to vitamin A in our bodies and helps boost healthy cell overturn. It also contains warming ginger and cinnamon to promote healthy circulation, which is important in creating a glowing complexion. The healthy fats it contains are also great for supporting supple, smooth skin.

1 cup peeled and sliced carrots

1 teaspoon peeled and minced fresh ginger

2 cups Fresh Hemp Milk (page 101), Fresh Almond Milk (page 100), or store-bought hemp or almond milk

2 medium frozen ripe bananas

¼ teaspoon ground cinnamon

In a blender, combine all the ingredients. Starting on low speed then increasing to high, blend the ingredients together until smooth.

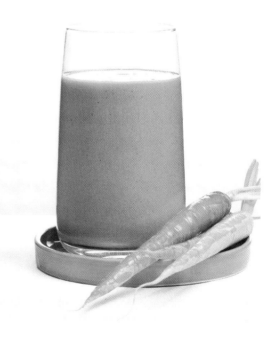

no-filter-needed-selfie smoothie

SERVES 2

What if you felt so great about yourself that you were okay posting pics without tweaks or filters? Well, we might not be totally filter-free all the time (including me for sure!), but we can drink our way to beautiful skin and higher natural energy as we work on all the deeper self-acceptance practices that we discussed in Part I. It's great to do both in tandem. This smoothie is loaded with vitamin C and healthy, nourishing beauty fats, as well as antioxidants and blood-purifying turmeric. Plus, it's delicious! Try it midmorning or during the afternoon, and just remember to drink it on an empty stomach for optimal digestion.

2 cups coconut water

1¾ cups fresh or frozen mango chunks

½ ripe avocado, pitted

1 tablespoon Chia Gel (page 104)

2 teaspoons vanilla extract

¼ teaspoon ground turmeric

1 tablespoon chopped fresh mint leaves

Pinch of sea salt

Combine all the ingredients in a blender. Starting on low speed, slowly increase the speed to high, and blend the ingredients together until smooth.

belly feel good smoothie

Papaya and pineapple possess enzymes and compounds such as bromelain that are fantastic for promoting excellent digestion. Ginger is also a great digestive aid, and aloe is soothing for your GI system. When we feel stressed and our stomach turns a bit, this is a great smoothie to help rebalance and feel good, starting in our bellies—because we know our bellies need to feel good for us to truly feel good!

2 cups diced fresh pineapple

2 cups peeled and diced fresh papaya

1 medium ripe banana

1½ cups coconut water

1 tablespoon fresh lime juice

½ teaspoon peeled and minced fresh ginger

1 teaspoon aloe juice

Pinch of sea salt

Combine all the ingredients in a blender. Starting on low speed, slowly increase the speed to high and blend the ingredients together until smooth, around 45 seconds.

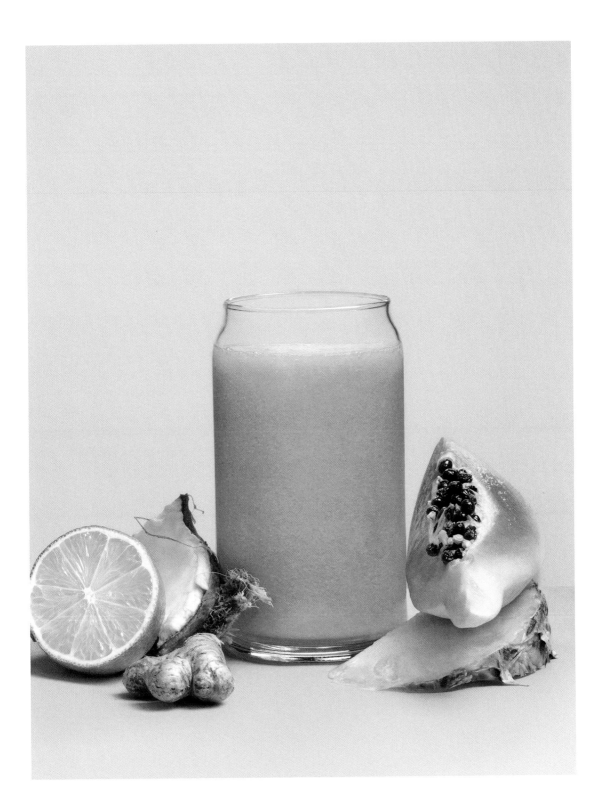

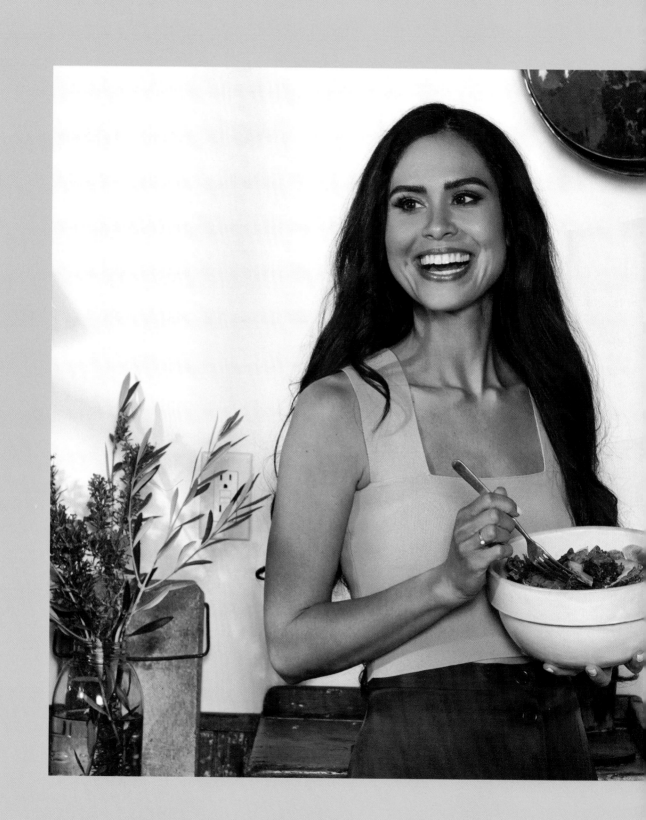

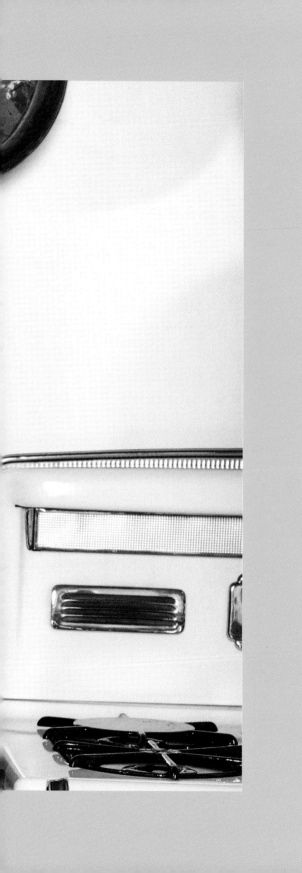

salads

Though we may know salads are good for us, we still need delicious, varied options in order to feel motivated to keep them a regular part of our lives. In the following salad recipes, my goal is to supply you with dishes that are as flavorful and fun to eat as they are good for you. Feel free, of course, to use these as a base, and tap your creative power to make your own happy, healthy versions!

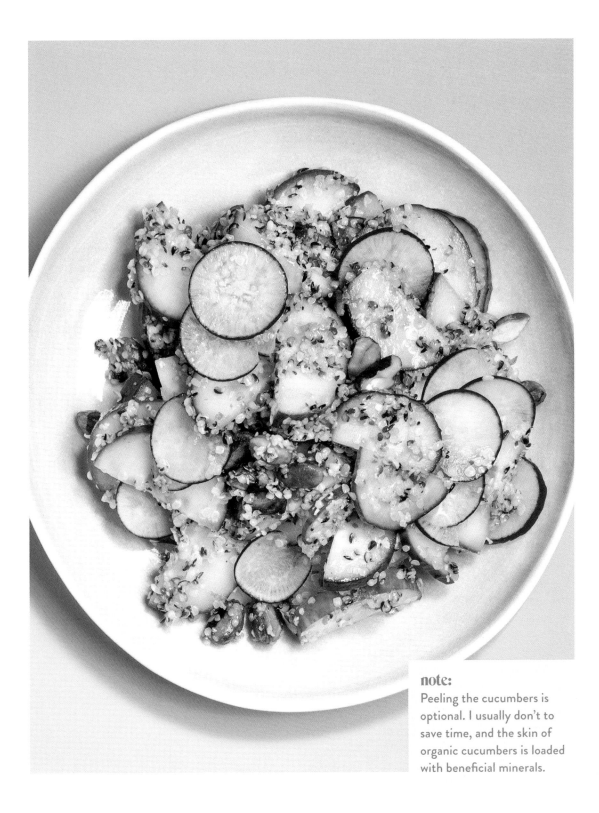

energizing pistachio hempseed cucumber salad
with orange zest

SERVES 4

Wow! This salad is so delicious and unique. It combines many interesting flavors you rarely enjoy all together. Just toss the ingredients and be prepared to be amazed at how incredibly alive you can feel from eating a salad! Food is such a powerful way to love yourself.

Hempseeds are a potent beauty food with skin-smoothing omega-3 fats and minerals, and pistachios are very high in protein.

2 cups hempseeds

3 cucumbers, cut in half lengthwise and sliced into ¼-inch pieces (see Note)

½ cup raw unsalted pistachios

5 radishes, thinly sliced

2 tablespoons olive oil

Grated zest and juice of 1 orange

Sea salt to taste

1. In a large bowl, toss the hempseeds, cucumbers, pistachios, and radishes together.

2. In a small bowl, mix together the olive oil, orange zest and juice, and sea salt.

3. Add the orange zest mixture to the hempseed and veggie mixture and toss to combine.

green power sprout salad
with creamy citrus dressing

SERVES 4

Sprouts are one of the biggest beauty and health foods secrets out there. They are so inexpensive most people overlook them. As if superfoods have to be expensive and rare—not so! Just as within all of us, there are treasures everywhere in nature.

Sprouts are "baby" plants and generate benefits for nearly every part of our bodies. They are bursting with nutrition, including protein, enzymes, fiber, manganese, riboflavin, copper, thiamin, niacin, pantothenic acid, iron, magnesium, potassium, and vitamins A, B_6, C, and K.

creamy citrus dressing

2 tablespoons pitted and mashed avocado

Juice of 1 small orange

1 tablespoon fresh lime juice

½ teaspoon sea salt

2 tablespoons olive oil

Freshly ground black pepper to taste

⅛ teaspoon cayenne pepper

1 green onion (scallion), white part and only 1 inch of green, coarsely chopped

salad

6 cups mixed greens or arugula

1 cup sunflower sprouts

1 cup clover or broccoli sprouts

2 radishes, thinly sliced

1. Make the creamy citrus dressing: In a small bowl, blend all the dressing ingredients together.

2. In a large bowl, toss the mixed greens, sprouts, and radishes together, then add the dressing and mix thoroughly with salad tongs or large spoons.

cucumber-tangerine salad

SERVES 4

Cucumbers are a wonderful food for radiant complexions, as they are hydrating and help flush toxins out while they supply electrolytes. The combination of all the ingredients in this salad is powerful and a great one to work into your rotation.

This salad provides an interesting citrus and Asian flavor combination. Sea vegetables supply trace minerals that complement land vegetables, so it's good to include them whenever possible. Nori is a sea vegetable packed with micronutrients, including vitamins B_{12} and C, as well as the minerals iron, calcium, and zinc.

2 medium cucumbers, thinly sliced

Sea salt

1 tablespoon tamari

1 tablespoon brown rice vinegar

1 teaspoon sesame oil

1 tangerine or orange, peeled and segmented

2 sheets nori seaweed, torn into 2-inch pieces

1 tablespoon black sesame seeds, for topping

1. Place the cucumber slices in a bowl. Sprinkle them with sea salt, massage it in, and leave for 15 minutes. Rinse the cucumbers, then using your hands, squeeze the cucumbers to drain them of any liquid.

2. In a separate bowl, mix together the tamari, brown rice vinegar, and sesame oil. Pour it over the cucumbers in the bowl, and toss with the citrus segments and nori pieces. Sprinkle the sesame seeds on top.

tempeh taco "meat" salad
with cashew sour cream

SERVES 4

This salad is complete enough to serve as a whole meal. It is both meat- and dairy-free yet has all the creamy and dense protein textures of a traditional Mexican salad. The deliciousness is there, with the added bonus that it's supportive to our bodies with plant-based protein, minerals, fiber, and more, and none of the congestive, blocking qualities. Now that is a supersalad!

cashew sour cream

1 cup raw unsalted cashews

¼ cup raw apple cider vinegar

½ teaspoon sea salt

salad

1 tablespoon coconut oil

8 ounces organic, non-GMO tempeh

2 teaspoons chili powder

¼ teaspoon dried oregano

1 teaspoon ground cumin

½ teaspoon paprika

¼ teaspoon cayenne pepper

¼ teaspoon freshly ground black pepper

2 romaine hearts, chopped

2 teaspoons fresh lemon juice

1 tablespoon olive oil

½ teaspoon sea salt

1 ripe tomato, quartered

1 avocado, pitted and sliced

1 large handful of fresh cilantro leaves

1. Make the cashew sour cream: In a blender, combine the cashews, cider vinegar, sea salt, and ⅓ cup of water, and blend on high speed until the mixture is smooth and creamy, about 1 minute; add a tablespoon or two of water if necessary. Refrigerate the dressing while making the rest of the dish (see Note).

2. In a skillet, melt the coconut oil over medium-high heat. Use your hands to crumble the tempeh into small pieces and add it to the skillet. Cook until it begins to brown, 5 to 7 minutes. Add the chili powder, oregano, and spices to the pan, along with ⅓ cup of water. Stir the mixture to evenly coat the tempeh with the spices. Continue to cook until the water is completely absorbed and the tempeh begins to brown and get crispy on the edges, 10 to 12 minutes.

3. While the tempeh cooks, toss the romaine in a bowl with the lemon juice, olive oil, sea salt, and tomato.

4. To serve, divide the salad evenly among four bowls, and top each with one-fourth of the tempeh mixture, avocado slices, and cilantro.

note:
There will be plenty of
cashew sour cream left
over—it's easier to blend a
larger quantity. Save it for
a veggie dip or even a
thicker salad dressing. It
will keep, refrigerated, for
up to 1 week.

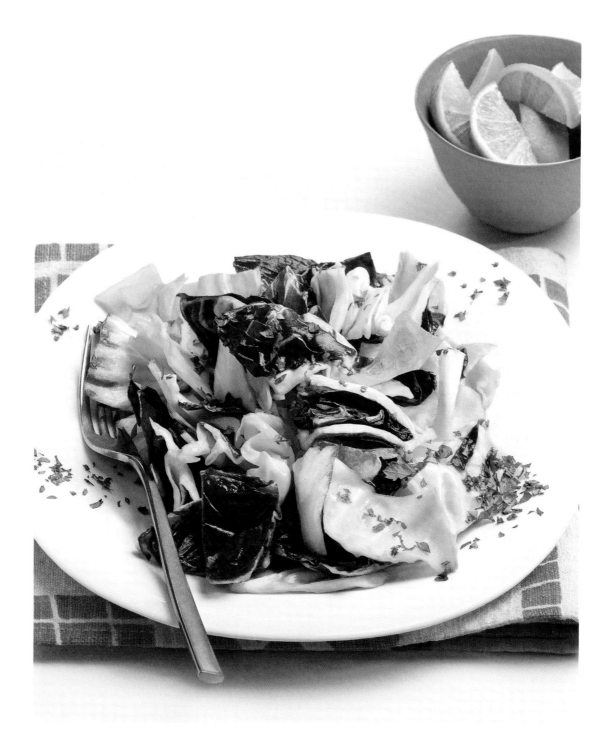

japanese super-cleanse salad

SERVES 2

This is inspired by one of my favorite Japanese restaurants in Los Angeles, called Shima, which happens to serve a lot of amazing vegan food. They have a similar salad on their menu, but it uses Japanese lime-like citrus fruit called yuzu. Yuzu has an exquisite taste yet is difficult to find, so instead we are doing our best by substituting regular limes in this recipe. This salad also stays crunchy for a few days, which is an added bonus, so you can make a larger batch and bring it to lunch the next day!

1 tablespoon fresh lime juice

1 tablespoon flax oil

1 tablespoon olive oil

½ teaspoon sea salt

1 head red radicchio, coarsely chopped into bite-size pieces

2 cups coarsely chopped bite-size pieces of green cabbage

2 tablespoons minced fresh parsley

1. In a small bowl, whisk the lime juice, flax oil, olive oil, and sea salt.

2. In a large serving bowl, toss the radicchio, green cabbage, and 1½ tablespoons of the parsley, and saturate the mixture with the dressing. Ideally, let it sit for at least 30 minutes before serving.

3. Sprinkle the last ½ tablespoon of parsley on top and around the edges of the bowl before serving.

kale, avocado, and grapefruit salad

SERVES 2

Eating whole grapefruit is detoxifying, as it is full of enzyme-rich water, fiber, and vitamins A and C, and it's known to be nourishing to the liver and kidneys, which are two organs responsible for cleansing your body of harmful substances.

I've been obsessed with kale salads since I started eating them with yogi friends back in New York City, where I lived upon coming back from my around-the-world trip. You might recall the Dharma's Kale Salad, now legendary in our community, from *The Beauty Detox Solution*. This new, exciting, yet simple version has a lot of freshness from the grapefruit and mint. A few awesome ingredients put together with loving care are often all it takes to make a really special dish!

2 teaspoons freshly squeezed orange juice

1 tablespoon olive oil

½ teaspoon sea salt

Freshly ground black pepper to taste

6 cups shredded lacinato kale leaves

1 pink grapefruit, peeled, sectioned, and cut into 2-inch pieces

1 avocado, pitted and sliced

2 tablespoons chopped fresh mint leaves

1. In a small bowl, combine the orange juice, olive oil, sea salt, and pepper for the dressing.

2. Place the kale in a large bowl and add all the dressing, massaging for a few minutes, until the leaves begin to break down a bit and become more tender.

3. Divide the kale between two plates. Top with the grapefruit and avocado. Sprinkle half of the mint on top of each serving.

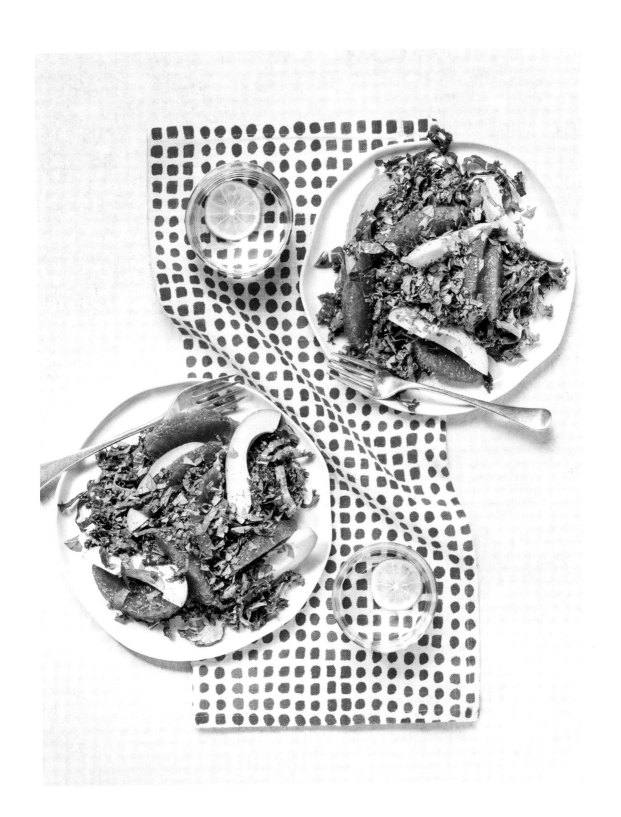

omega-arugula salad
with pecans and lime vinaigrette

Bitter foods are one of the important tastes to eat according to Ayurveda, but in the Western world, we often miss out on them. Bitter greens help support our livers, purify our blood, cleanse our systems, help our skin glow, and improve digestion. They have a bold flavor that is balanced in this recipe with the richness of pecans, a top antioxidant-containing food. Pecans are also an incredible source of beauty- and health-enhancing nutrients, including folate, calcium, magnesium, phosphorus, potassium, zinc, antioxidants, and vitamins A, B, and E.

Since this salad is so balancing, it's great to eat when you feel a little out of balance, which we all do from time to time.

salad

- 5 ounces arugula (I love wild arugula, if you can find it)
- 1 carrot, peeled into ribbons
- ½ cup coarsely chopped pecans

lime vinaigrette

- 1½ tablespoons flax oil or olive oil (see Note)
- 2 teaspoons fresh lime juice
- 1 teaspoon coconut nectar
- ¼ teaspoon freshly ground black pepper
- Sea salt to taste

1. In a large bowl, toss together the arugula, carrot, and pecans.

2. Make the lime vinaigrette: In a small bowl, mix the oil, lime juice, coconut nectar, pepper, and sea salt. Pour over the salad, toss, and enjoy fresh!

note:

I like using raw flax oil, as it contains essential omega fats that are not found in olive oil (which is made up of monounsaturated fats). Omega-3 fats are necessary for hormonal, skin, and heart health, and more. It's a bit pricey, but if you can swing it (at least sometimes), I think it's a good health investment. Be sure to keep it in the fridge to prevent it from going rancid.

asian sesame dressing

While true beauty is really about the overall vibration we put into the world, we still care about the state of our skin—and there is nothing at all wrong with that! Sesame oil is believed to improve the health of our hair and skin. Sesame seeds are a strengthening food, a rich source of calcium and other minerals. It's important to rotate in tasty salad dressings to keep us excited to eat our life-supporting greens.

1 tablespoon sesame seeds

3 tablespoons brown rice vinegar

¼ cup avocado oil or olive oil

2 tablespoons sesame oil

1 tablespoon tamari

2 teaspoons coconut sugar

Grind the sesame seeds in a mortar and pestle or spice grinder. Place them in a small bowl, add the rest of the ingredients, and whisk to combine. Store in an airtight container in the refrigerator for 1 to 2 weeks.

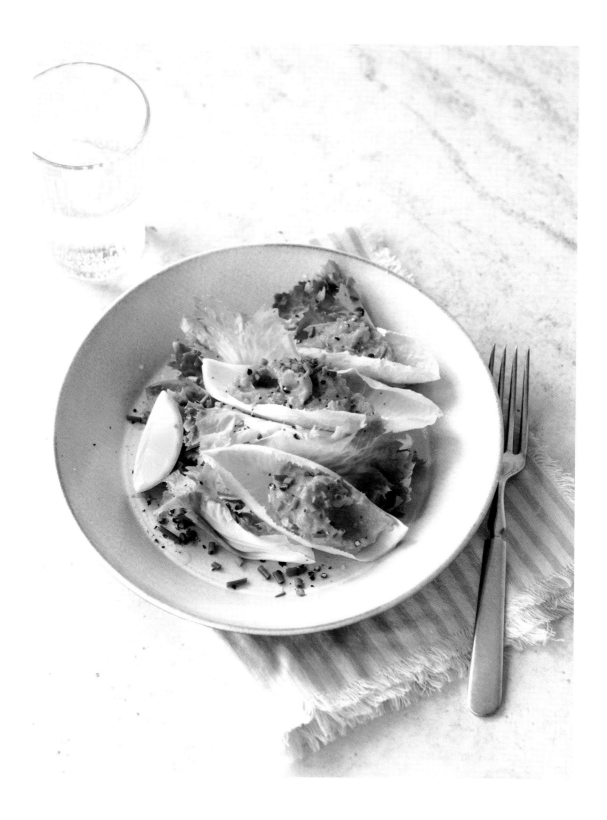

endive, escarole, and creamy sweet potato salad

SERVES 4

Besides supplying a lot of rich nutrients, including vitamins C and K and folate, this salad is assembled in a stacked, festive way that is fun to eat and serve. Endive leaves are a perfect "boat" for holding the sweet potato mix.

2 medium sweet potatoes (about ¾ pound total)

3 tablespoons coconut yogurt

1 teaspoon raw apple cider vinegar

1 teaspoon olive oil

1 teaspoon Dijon mustard

1 tablespoon fresh thyme leaves, or 1 teaspoon dried

Sea salt

Freshly ground black pepper to taste

1 head escarole, chopped

Juice of 1 lemon

1 head endive, trimmed and leaves separated

1 tablespoon minced fresh chives, for garnish

1. Preheat the oven to 375°F.

2. Pierce the sweet potatoes all over and then bake on a baking sheet until softened, about 45 minutes or so. Set aside to cool.

3. Meanwhile, in a bowl, whisk together the coconut yogurt, cider vinegar, oil, mustard, thyme, ¼ teaspoon sea salt, and pepper for the dressing.

4. When the sweet potatoes are cool enough to handle, cut them in half lengthwise and scoop the flesh into the bowl of dressing, folding everything together gently. Mash the potatoes a bit, but retain some chunky texture.

5. Arrange the escarole on four plates. Drizzle the lemon juice over the escarole and season with sea salt and pepper. Place 2 or 3 endive leaves on top of each plate and scoop some of the potato salad into each leaf. Garnish the endive–potato salad mixture with the chives.

earth lover's mustard-maple dressing

MAKES ABOUT ⅓ CUP

I don't usually like dressings with sweetness, yet recently, when traveling in Chile, I discovered a healthy café that offered many different salads, all of which were made with sweet dressings (the chef there used molasses as the sweetener). The sweetness paired with the greens felt good in my body, and there is a time and a place for such dressings. So I offer this sweet recipe for when you want to feel pacified or soothed. When the outer world is feeling a bit chaotic, sometimes we just want to feel a little sweet inside!

3 tablespoons
maple syrup

2 teaspoons raw apple
cider vinegar

2 tablespoons Dijon
mustard

3 tablespoons olive oil

½ teaspoon sea salt

Freshly ground black
pepper to taste

In a small bowl, whisk all the ingredients together. Store in an airtight container in the refrigerator for up to 1 week.

beautifying thousand island dressing

MAKES ABOUT ½ CUP

I have had clients who grew up eating Thousand Island dressing and were quite attached to it. This version is a pretty awesome replacement, I have to say, and without mayonnaise. I tested it on some traditional Thousand Island lovers, and they all told me it was pretty darn close! So if you or someone in your life is a Thousand Island fan, you'll be pretty excited about this noncongestive yet tasty version.

8 ounces organic, non-GMO silken tofu

1½ tablespoons brown rice vinegar

1½ tablespoons avocado oil or olive oil

1 tablespoon coconut nectar or maple syrup

1 tablespoon organic ketchup

2 teaspoons organic pickle relish

1 teaspoon sea salt, or to taste

⅛ teaspoon freshly ground black pepper

⅛ teaspoon mustard powder

In a small bowl, whisk all the ingredients together. Store in an airtight container in the refrigerator for up to 1 week.

bounty earth salad

As its name indicates, this salad feels like you're eating the earth. And the combination of all kinds of potatoes with greens unites the qualities of earthy and light. Yin and yang. Remember our "and" principle (see page 15)? All things can be many things at one time . . . including in our recipes!

salad

1 small sweet potato (about ¼ pound), cubed

2 small purple potatoes, cubed

1 russet potato (about ½ pound), cubed

1 tablespoon coconut oil, melted

6 cups mixed salad greens

dressing

3 tablespoons olive oil

1 teaspoon raw apple cider vinegar

¼ teaspoon sea salt

1 tablespoon Dijon mustard

2 teaspoons balsamic vinegar

Freshly ground black pepper to taste

1 teaspoon chopped fresh tarragon

1. Preheat the oven to 425°F.

2. In a bowl, toss the potatoes with the coconut oil. Place them in a single layer on a baking sheet. Roast until tender, about 30 minutes.

3. Meanwhile, make the dressing: Whisk all the dressing ingredients together in a small bowl until mixed thoroughly.

4. In a serving bowl, toss the dressing with the roasted veggies, then add the greens, toss, and let them wilt.

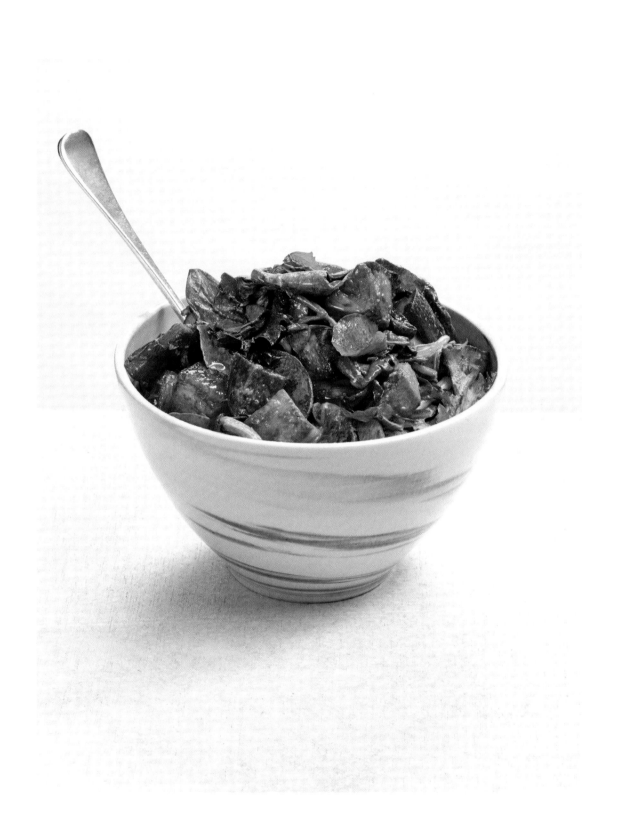

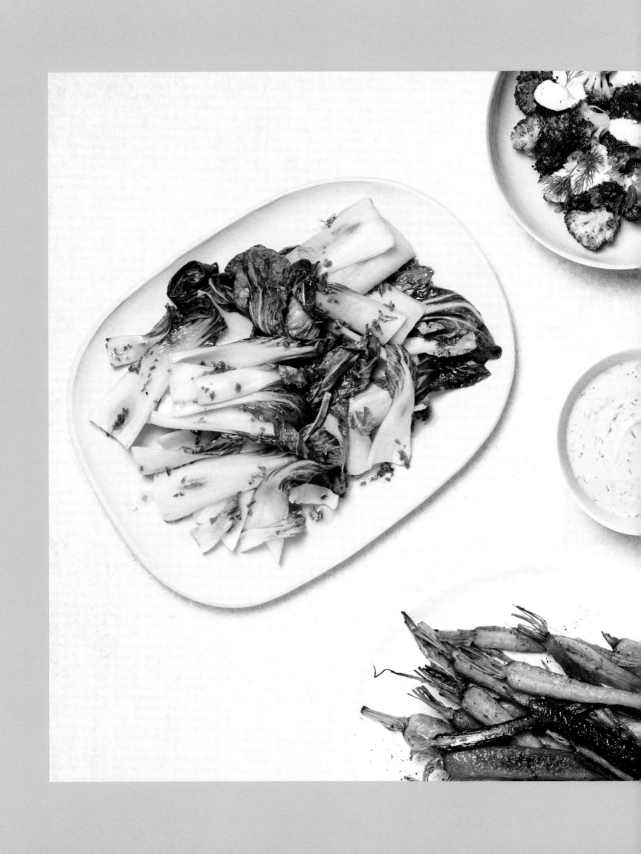

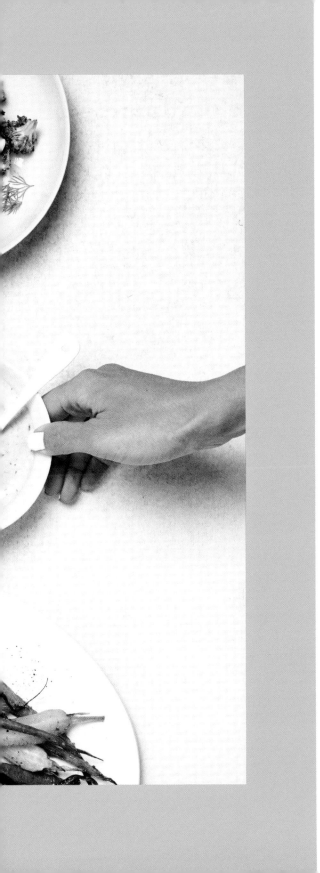

starters and side dishes

To round out our lifestyle, we also need great options to start our meals and to serve alongside our entrées, salads, and soups. This section has so many delicious options that are cleansing and support vitality.

Many of these sides, eaten in larger portion sizes, are nutritionally complete enough to be made into mains for lunch or dinner. Try some first that call out to you, then adventure into experimenting with others. As with all things in life, we are often very pleasantly surprised when we let go of our comfort zone and explore beyond!

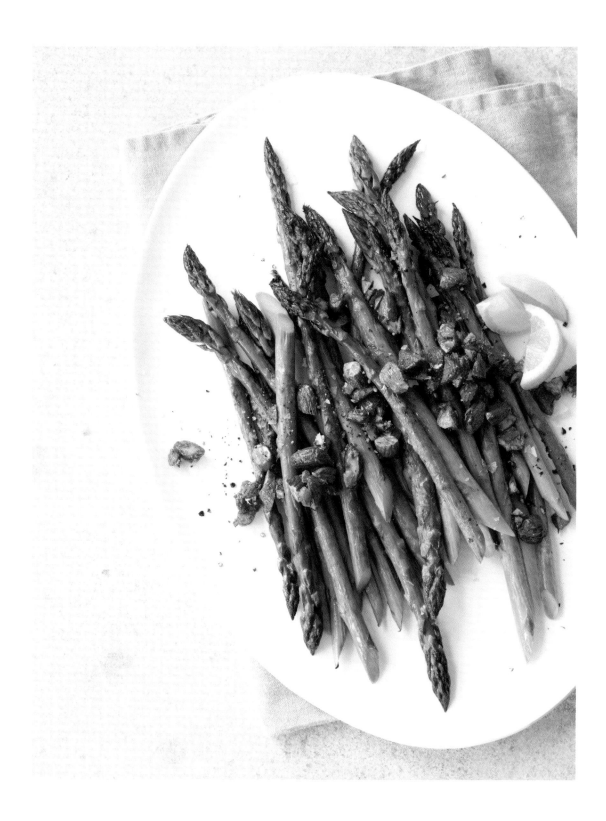

asparagus
with spicy almonds

SERVES 2 TO 4

Almonds and other nuts are usually best eaten raw to preserve their delicate oils and amino acids. But in the spirit of perfectly imperfect, sometimes it's okay to heat them up. And it's delicious! Heating will not alter the wonderful mix of minerals, which include magnesium, copper, and calcium, as well as vitamin E. Asparagus is high in vitamin K and fiber; it also is a natural diuretic.

These two beautiful ingredients create a delicious, nutritious combination.

2 teaspoons coconut oil, melted, plus more for greasing

1 tablespoon coconut nectar or maple syrup

½ teaspoon cayenne pepper

¼ teaspoon ground turmeric

Sea salt

½ cup sliced or chopped almonds

1 pound asparagus, ends removed

Freshly ground black pepper to taste

1 tablespoon fresh lemon juice

1. Preheat the oven to 350°F. Grease a baking sheet and a 9-inch square glass baking dish with some coconut oil.

2. In a small mixing bowl, combine the coconut nectar, cayenne pepper, turmeric, and ¼ teaspoon sea salt. Add the almonds and mix them around until evenly coated. Spread the almonds on the prepared baking sheet. Set it to the side.

3. Place the asparagus in a single layer in the prepared baking dish (it's okay if some get stacked), coat the asparagus with the 2 teaspoons coconut oil, and season with sea salt and black pepper.

4. Place the almonds and asparagus in the oven. Bake both for about 10 minutes, stirring each about halfway through. If a more tender texture for the asparagus is desired, leave for 5 more minutes.

5. Remove the almonds and asparagus from the oven and transfer the asparagus to a serving dish. Sprinkle the almonds over the asparagus, and drizzle fresh lemon juice on top.

sweet cleanse turmeric-roasted root veggies

SERVES 6

Roasted root veggies are grounding and comforting. When we practice grounding, or walking barefoot on the earth's surface, we get some healing simply by being in contact with the earth's energy field and the negative ions it gives off, which help protect us from free radicals. And when we eat directly from the earth, we also reconnect, especially with veggies that are grown within the earth itself.

This roasted dish also contains the magical spice turmeric, which cleanses the blood and helps reduce inflammation.

¼ cup coconut oil, melted, plus more for greasing

4 medium carrots, cut into 1-inch slices

1 medium acorn or butternut squash, peeled, seeded, and cut into 1-inch cubes

2 medium red beets, peeled and cut into 1-inch cubes

2 sweet potatoes or yams, cut into 1-inch cubes

1 teaspoon sea salt

2 tablespoons coconut nectar

1 teaspoon ground turmeric

½ teaspoon ground cinnamon

1. Preheat the oven to 375°F. Grease a 9 × 13-inch glass baking dish or rimmed baking sheet.

2. In a large bowl, toss together the carrots, squash, beets, and sweet potatoes with the coconut oil.

3. In a small bowl, mix together the sea salt, coconut nectar, turmeric, and cinnamon, and toss over the veggies.

4. Spread the veggies in the prepared baking dish and bake until tender, about 1 hour, stirring halfway through.

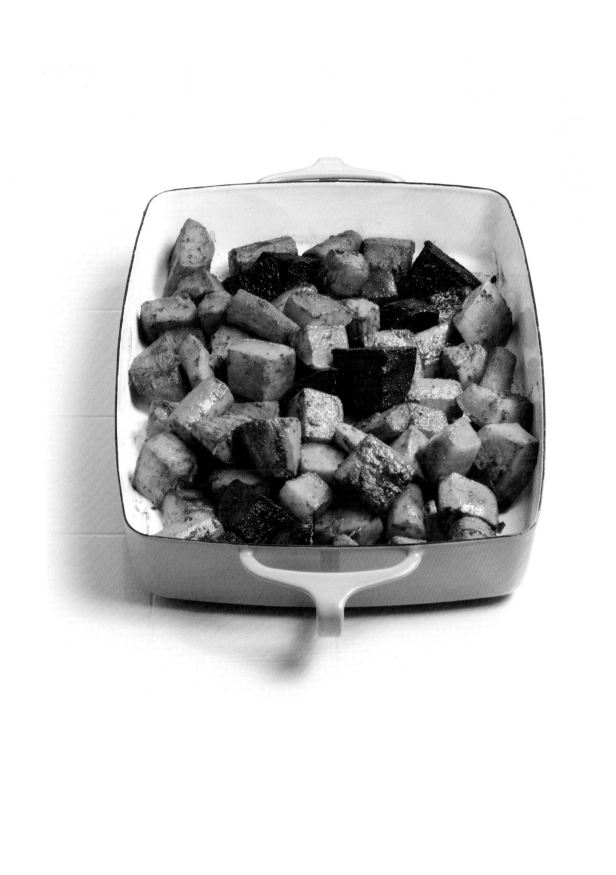

kgfm fennel casserole

SERVES 6

I thought I would have fun with this name, simply because life should be fun and we don't need to take anything too seriously. It's short for "Kim's Gluten-Free Mushroom and Fennel Casserole." Sure, you have to clean up the food processor, but once you stuff the casserole in the oven, it's smooth sailing, with no stirring or nada left to do. The joys of oven cooking!

Fennel is a cleansing food high in fiber, potassium, folate, vitamin C, vitamin B_6, and phytonutrients. It also contains selenium, which contributes to liver enzyme function and helps detoxify the body.

6 slices gluten-free bread

Coconut oil, melted, for greasing

2 fennel bulbs, trimmed, cored, and thinly sliced lengthwise

1 cup sliced oyster mushrooms or cremini mushrooms

2 medium carrots, sliced

1½ cups coconut milk

Juice of 1 lemon

3 tablespoons coarsely chopped fresh sage leaves

Sea salt and freshly ground black pepper to taste

¼ cup coarsely chopped fresh basil or parsley leaves, for garnish

1. Preheat the oven to 375°F.

2. Place the gluten-free bread on a baking sheet and toast until it is lightly browned, about 8 minutes, flipping the slices halfway through. Set aside, but leave the oven on. Once it has cooled, process the toast into crumbs using a food processor.

3. Grease an 8-inch square glass baking dish or a Dutch oven. Add the fennel, mushrooms, carrots, coconut milk, lemon juice, sage, and bread crumbs to the prepared baking dish and toss. Season with sea salt and pepper. Bake, uncovered, for 30 to 35 minutes, until the top is toasty and browned. Garnish with the chopped basil.

tangy cranberry parsnip "rice"

Though most of us may not use parsnips as often as other veggies, they have an interesting flavor and contain earthy, strengthening qualities, like other root veggies, and nutrients such as fiber, vitamin C, and folate. Combined with the astringent taste of the cranberry, this dish offers a tart balance alongside other dishes, especially creamy ones. Cranberries are a detoxifying food and a great source of antioxidants and phytonutrients. Try to use unsweetened cranberries, although they may be hard to find (if you have to use cranberries that are sweetened with some kind of sugar, don't sweat it—the amount of sugar per serving won't be much).

2 parsnips, peeled

1 cup cauliflower florets

1½ tablespoons olive oil

2 tablespoons fresh lemon juice (from about 1 lemon)

⅓ cup dried cranberries

2 teaspoons coconut sugar

1 teaspoon sea salt

Freshly ground black pepper to taste

Combine all the ingredients in a food processor and process until finely chopped, about 1 minute.

note:
There will be plenty of extra tzatziki sauce, which can be used as a salad dressing or a topping for steamed or roasted vegetables later in the week. We have to make more for easier blending purposes! It will keep in an airtight container for up to 5 days in the fridge.

roasted broccoli
with pine nut tzatziki sauce

SERVES 4

Pine nuts are a true beauty food delicacy. They are sourced from the mighty stone pine, *Pinus pinea,* and the nuts take between eighteen months and three years to grow, making them a treasure when they are finally harvested. They nourish us with antioxidants, lutein, and vitamins A, B, C, D, and E. They also make a fantastic creamy texture replacement for dairy. Broccoli is a great source of protein (yes, green veggies can be a great source!), folate, vitamins K and C, and so much more.

Combining these two ingredients, you'll get a powerful dish as a side, or, with a larger portion size, a nourishing entrée.

roasted broccoli

3 medium heads broccoli (about 2 pounds total), cut into florets

2 tablespoons coconut oil, melted, plus more for greasing

Sea salt and freshly ground black pepper to taste

pine nut tzatziki sauce

¼ cup pine nuts

½ cup raw unsalted cashews

2 tablespoons fresh lemon juice

⅔ cup coconut milk

2 tablespoons minced white onion

Pinch of sea salt

2 tablespoons minced fresh dill leaves

2 tablespoons minced fresh mint leaves

1. Preheat the oven to 400°F.

2. In a bowl, toss the broccoli with the 2 tablespoons coconut oil and lightly season it with sea salt and pepper. Grease a baking sheet with coconut oil and spread the broccoli on top. Roast for 20 minutes.

3. Meanwhile, make the pine nut tzatziki sauce: In a blender or food processor, blend the pine nuts, cashews, lemon juice, coconut milk, onion, and sea salt until smooth and creamy, 30 to 45 seconds. Stir in 1 tablespoon each of the minced dill and mint.

4. To serve, arrange the broccoli on a serving dish and pour some of the sauce over the top (see Note). Top with the remaining dill and mint.

roasted brussels sprouts
with tahini special sauce

SERVES 4

Creamy textures can feel luscious and soothing for the soul. The key is to make sure we create the creaminess from the bounty of plant-based options rather than from dairy, so we feel good and light. The star ingredients of this protein- and calcium-rich dish are Brussels sprouts and restorative tahini. The pine nuts add extra crunch.

roasted brussels sprouts

2 tablespoons coconut oil, melted, plus more for greasing

4 pounds Brussels sprouts, trimmed and halved lengthwise

Sea salt and freshly ground black pepper to taste

tahini special sauce

¼ cup tahini

¼ cup fresh lemon juice

½ teaspoon sea salt

2 tablespoons dried cranberries or raisins

¼ cup minced fresh parsley

2 tablespoons black sesame seeds

⅓ cup pine nuts

1. Preheat the oven to 375°F. Grease a 9 × 13-inch baking dish with coconut oil.

2. In a large bowl, toss the Brussels sprouts with the 2 tablespoons of coconut oil, sea salt, and pepper. Spread the Brussels sprouts evenly in the prepared baking dish. Place a pan of water on the bottom shelf of the oven to prevent the sprouts from drying out. Roast for 30 minutes, or until browned and softened.

3. Meanwhile, make the tahini special sauce: In a food processor or blender, combine the tahini, lemon juice, sea salt, and 2 tablespoons water, and process until smooth and creamy. Set to the side.

4. Arrange the roasted sprouts on a serving platter. Drizzle the sauce over the top, then top with the cranberries, parsley, black sesame seeds, and pine nuts.

protein rolls
with aioli-soy dipping sauce

**MAKES 12 HALF
HANDHELD ROLLS**

Sushi rolls are so much fun to eat. We don't all get to eat sea vegetables every day, and their slightly ocean-y taste is unique. I had a quinoa sushi roll recipe in *The Beauty Detox Power*, and I wanted to try a protein twist version of it, using organic tofu (see page 85 for more info on soy). These rolls are quick to make and delicious to eat on the go, sans rice or any kind of starch. The sauce is so good it can even be used as a dip or salad dressing. Try it for yourself!

protein rolls

6 standard nori sheets

4 ounces organic, non-GMO firm tofu, cut into ¼-inch-thick strips

1 carrot, cut into matchsticks

1½ cups broccoli sprouts

aioli-soy dipping sauce

½ cup raw unsalted cashews

2 tablespoons coconut milk

1 tablespoon coconut nectar or maple syrup

1 teaspoon raw apple cider vinegar

2 tablespoons tamari

2 teaspoons olive oil

1 tablespoon minced fresh chives

1 tablespoon minced fresh tarragon

1. To make the protein rolls, lay the nori sheets flat, and line one short end of each with a fourth of the tofu, carrot, and broccoli sprouts. Roll up the nori very tightly, moisten the ends with some water, and press firmly to close (see my Facebook Live Cooking Show [#kimcookslive] demo for this rolling technique). Holding a sharp kitchen knife at an angle, pierce the nori wrapper to make an initial slit, then cut each nori wrapper crosswise in half.

2. Make the aioli-soy dipping sauce: In a blender or food processor blend the cashews, coconut milk, coconut nectar, cider vinegar, tamari, and oil until smooth. Place the mixture in a bowl and stir in the chives and tarragon. Serve immediately with the rolls.

lightness green cuke rolls

MAKES ABOUT 9 ROLLS

These all-veggie rolls are pretty to serve and full of healthy fat, B vitamins, minerals such as calcium, and more. The only thing is . . . you must eat these rolls almost immediately! Roll and eat is best, before the cukes start getting soggy. Food that you can pick up with your hands is fun and helps put you back directly in touch with your food.

1 avocado, pitted

¼ cup fresh basil leaves

2 teaspoons fresh lemon juice

¼ teaspoon sea salt

1 tablespoon nutritional yeast

1 medium cucumber, unpeeled

1 tablespoon black sesame seeds

1. In a blender or food processor, combine the avocado, basil, lemon juice, sea salt, and nutritional yeast and blend until smooth, 20 to 30 seconds. Transfer to a small bowl. Set to the side.

2. Using a mandoline, cut the cucumber lengthwise into long, thin strips.

3. Spread about 2 teaspoons of the avocado mixture along the length of a cucumber strip. Make sure to get some avocado all the way to the end, so the roll will stick together. Sprinkle it with about ¼ teaspoon of the sesame seeds.

4. Tightly roll the cucumber strip up. Repeat with the remaining strips.

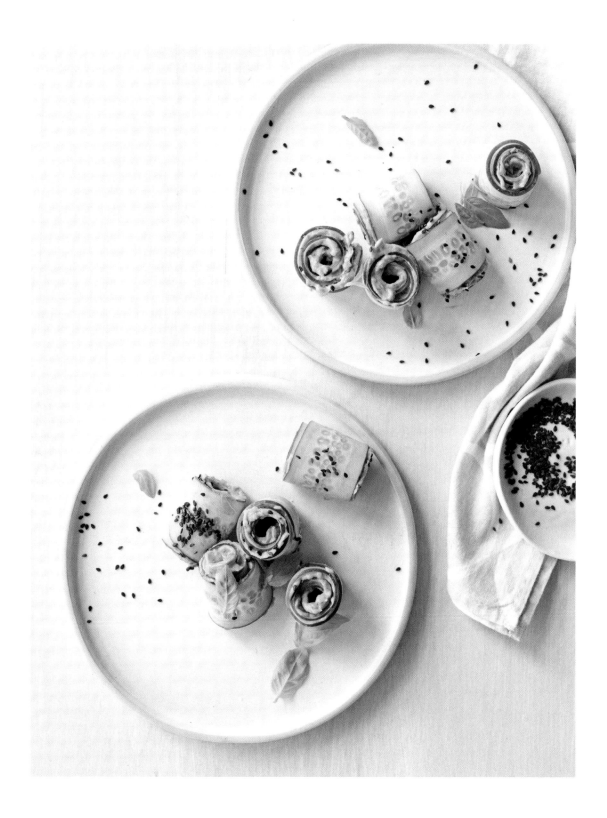

steamed veggies
with miso mustard sauce

SERVES 4

I am obsessed with Japan and so many things about it, including their artful way of preparing food. I had such beautiful food there, including the temple cuisine, or *shojin ryori,* which is served at Zen Buddhist temples and certain restaurants. I was able to find plenty of great plant foods, including artisanally prepared tofu, a wide variety of mushrooms, and miso sauces such as the one featured here. Miso is nutritious fermented food, and paired with steamed veggies, it makes a beautiful and balanced dish.

steamed veggies

4 carrots, cut into 2-inch pieces

1 cup broccoli florets

1 cup cauliflower florets

1 small head bok choy (about 1 pound), root ends cut so leaves separate individually

mustard miso sauce

¼ cup mellow white miso paste

3 tablespoons Dijon mustard

3 tablespoons coconut nectar or maple syrup

1. Place a steamer basket in the bottom of a pot, and fill the pot with water to just below the level of the basket. Place all the veggies in the basket and bring the water to a boil. Reduce the heat to medium-low, cover the pot, and simmer for about 9 minutes, until the veggies have softened.

2. Meanwhile, make the mustard miso sauce: Whisk all the sauce ingredients together. Serve in a bowl to the side of the steamed veggies for spreading or dipping.

ayurvedic-inspired mushroom gravy

SERVES 4

This is a rich, gravy-like sauce that can be served with the Lentil Love Loaf (page 204), steamed or roasted veggies, or whatever else you might like. This recipe is full of the warming spices cinnamon, cloves, coriander, and turmeric, which are classically used in Ayurvedic cooking.

Oyster mushrooms have a rich three-thousand-year history in Traditional Chinese Medicine, particularly as a tonic for the immune system. They also contain significant levels of zinc, iron, potassium, calcium, phosphorus, vitamin C, folic acid, niacin, and vitamins B_1 (thiamine) and B_2 (riboflavin).

1 tablespoon olive oil

¼ cup chopped yellow onions

2½ cups sliced oyster mushrooms

¾ cup coconut milk

½ teaspoon ground cinnamon

5 whole cloves

2 teaspoons ground coriander

¼ teaspoon ground turmeric

1 teaspoon sea salt

1. In a large pan, heat the olive oil and cook the onions, softening them. Add the mushrooms and cook through for 3 to 4 minutes, until softened.

2. Transfer the onions and mushrooms to a blender. Add the coconut milk, cinnamon, cloves, coriander, turmeric, sea salt, and ⅓ cup of water; blend for 30 to 45 seconds, until smooth, or, if you prefer a slightly chunkier gravy, for only 20 to 30 seconds.

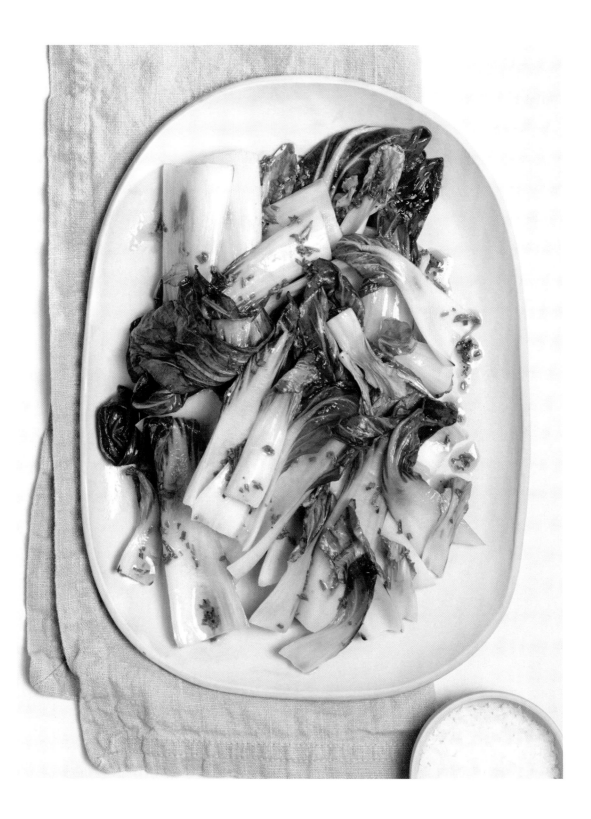

strengthening warm bok choy
with rosemary dressing

SERVES 2 TO 4

Bok choy is a powerhouse, vitality-supporting food that is common in China and Japan. However, those of us in the West usually don't consume it as much, though hopefully this delicious recipe will inspire you to seek it out more. Bok choy also contains vitamins A, C, and K, and is an excellent source of minerals such as calcium, magnesium, potassium, manganese, and iron.

1 tablespoon coconut oil

4 heads baby bok choy, root ends removed so that leaves separate individually

¼ cup flax oil or olive oil

1 tablespoon fresh lemon juice

1 tablespoon coconut nectar

2 teaspoons chopped fresh rosemary

½ teaspoon sea salt, or to taste

Freshly ground black pepper to taste

2 tablespoons pine nuts, for garnish

1. In a saucepan, melt the coconut oil over medium-high heat. Add the bok choy leaves and sauté for 3 to 5 minutes, until the greens are wilted and the stalks are crisp-tender.

2. Meanwhile, in a small bowl, whisk the flax oil, lemon juice, coconut nectar, rosemary, sea salt, and pepper together until thoroughly combined.

3. Arrange the bok choy on a serving plate, drizzle evenly with the dressing, and top with the pine nuts.

kale and sesame seed slaw

SERVES 1 OR 2

Kale is a veggie high in fiber, amino acids that build protein and contribute to overall strength, and minerals such as calcium and iron. It also contains B vitamins and vitamin C, which we need for non-heme, plant-based iron absorption. Sesame seeds also happen to be an incredible source of calcium and iron as well, making this recipe a mineral-dense supercombination.

1 bunch kale (about 1 pound)

1 large carrot (about ¼ pound), shredded

1 tablespoon olive oil

1 tablespoon fresh lemon juice

Sea salt and freshly ground black pepper to taste

2 tablespoons white sesame seeds

Grated zest of 1 orange

1. Remove the tough rib or vein of each leaf of kale and shred the leaves as finely as possible. Place in a large bowl, add the grated carrot, and mix.

2. In a small bowl, mix together the oil, lemon juice, sea salt, and pepper. Toss the dressing with the kale and carrots. Adjust the seasonings if needed.

3. Sprinkle the sesame seeds and orange zest on top.

creamy eggplant rounds

SERVES 4

This is a fun dish to serve at the beginning of a meal or as a side dish to your main, with a few beautifully arranged pieces served to each person. Coconut yogurt can commonly be found today in many markets. It contains some healthy probiotic bacteria (though no yogurt has a range of strains that can replace an excellent probiotic supplement), is dairy-free, and digests well.

3 tablespoons
coconut oil

1 medium eggplant
(about 1½ pounds),
peeled and sliced
crosswise into
¼-inch-thick rounds

Sea salt and freshly
ground black pepper
to taste

1 cup balsamic vinegar

⅓ cup chopped fresh
basil leaves

coconut-aioli sauce

½ cup unsweetened
plain coconut yogurt

2 teaspoons fresh lime
juice

1 teaspoon olive oil

½ teaspoon minced
fresh parsley

¼ teaspoon sea salt

Freshly ground black
pepper to taste

1. In a large skillet, melt the coconut oil over medium heat. Working in batches, add the eggplant rounds and cook until they are browned on each side, about 5 minutes each. Transfer the rounds to paper towels to soak up the excess oil. Season with sea salt and pepper.

2. Place the balsamic vinegar in a small saucepan and simmer over medium-low heat until the vinegar has reduced by half the original amount; it should take 10 to 15 minutes for 1 cup of vinegar to reduce to ½ cup.

3. In a small bowl, whisk together the coconut-aioli sauce ingredients until mixed thoroughly.

4. Arrange the eggplant rounds on a serving platter. Using a small spoon, top each with a drizzle of the balsamic reduction, about 2 teaspoons of the coconut-aioli sauce, and some fresh basil leaves.

awesome vegan (av) stuffing

SERVES 8

This is a hearty, rejuvenating dish made with gluten-free bread; I like brown-rice or millet-based gluten-free bread. And definitely source fresh herbs for this—it's worth it. This is so good you won't want to save stuffing only for the holidays!

6 slices gluten-free bread

3 tablespoons coconut oil, plus more for greasing

½ cup diced white onion

1 cup diced carrots

1 cup diced celery

1½ cups chopped cremini mushrooms

1 tablespoon minced fresh rosemary

2 teaspoons fresh thyme leaves

2 teaspoons minced fresh sage

2 cups vegetable broth

Sea salt and freshly ground black pepper to taste

1. Preheat the oven to 375°F.

2. Place the gluten-free bread on a baking sheet and toast it until browned, about 10 minutes, flipping the slices halfway through. Remove from the oven and set aside to cool, but leave the oven on. When the bread has cooled, cut it into ½-inch pieces. (Note: Stack the bread, and you can do this pretty quickly.)

3. Meanwhile, in a saucepan, heat the 3 tablespoons coconut oil and sauté the onion, carrots, celery, mushrooms, rosemary, thyme, and sage until the veggies have lightly softened, about 5 minutes. Stir in the vegetable broth.

4. Add the bread pieces to the pan and season with salt and pepper. Grease a 9 × 9-inch glass baking dish. Place the mixture in the prepared baking dish and bake, covered, for 30 minutes. Uncover and bake for 10 more minutes, or until the top is lightly browned.

carrot, red lentil, and walnut dip

MAKES ¾ CUP

This is a fantastically restorative, nutritious dip to pair with veggies. Lentils are a great source of protein, while skin-nurturing and brain-power-boosting walnuts provide plant-based omega-3s, vitamin E, and folate. Since legumes food combine (see page 84 for more info) both as a starch and a protein, here we are combining them as a protein.

2 medium carrots (about ½ pound total), cut into 2-inch pieces

2 teaspoons coconut oil, melted

1 teaspoon curry powder

¼ cup uncooked red lentils, thoroughly rinsed

1 cup filtered water

1 tablespoon walnut pieces

1 tablespoon olive oil

¼ cup chopped fresh cilantro leaves, plus more for garnish

2 tablespoons tahini

2½ tablespoons fresh lemon juice

¾ teaspoon ground coriander

½ teaspoon ground cumin

⅛ teaspoon cayenne pepper

Sea salt

Freshly ground black pepper to taste

Chopped fresh parsley, for garnish (optional)

1. Preheat the oven to 400°F.

2. Place the carrots on a baking sheet, drizzle with the coconut oil, and sprinkle with the curry powder. Roast the carrots in the oven for 25 to 30 minutes, until fork-tender and golden brown, tossing them about halfway through.

3. Meanwhile, combine the lentils and filtered water in a medium saucepan over high heat. Bring to a boil, reduce the heat, and simmer, uncovered, for 10 to 15 minutes, until tender, stirring occasionally. Drain off any excess water.

4. Add the roasted carrots, walnuts, olive oil, and cooked lentils to a food processor, along with the ¼ cup cilantro, the tahini, lemon juice, coriander, cumin, cayenne, ¾ teaspoon sea salt (or to taste), and pepper. Process until smooth. Scrape into a serving bowl and garnish with the chopped parsley and remaining cilantro. Serve with fresh veggies.

apple creek ranch ginger-roasted carrots

SERVES 2 TO 4

We shot the cover and many of the lifestyle photos for this book at my friend Todd's beautiful Apple Creek Ranch, from which Sunrise Organic Farm operates, located in northern Santa Barbara County. They grow the most amazingly tasty carrots. We all noshed on them right out of the ground during the shoot. It helped inspire this warming, beta-carotene-rich recipe.

1 tablespoon coconut oil, melted, plus more for greasing

2 pounds carrots (around 10 carrots), sliced in half lengthwise and horizontally

1 (1½-inch) piece of ginger, peeled and grated

¼ teaspoon ground cinnamon

Sea salt and freshly ground black pepper to taste

1. Preheat the oven to 400°F. Grease a 9 × 13-inch glass baking dish with coconut oil.

2. In the prepared baking dish, toss the carrots with the ginger, the 1 tablespoon coconut oil, the cinnamon, and sea salt and pepper. Roast for about 40 minutes, or until the carrots are tender to your liking, stirring partway through.

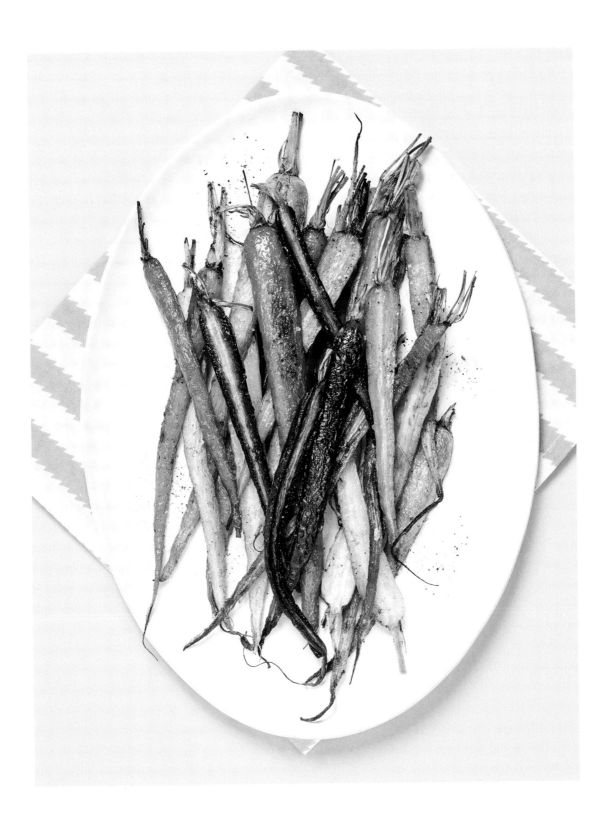

creamy spinach and dill hummus
with pine nuts

MAKES 1 CUP

This creamy hummus features dill, a food that supports our happiness, with some research in the *American Journal of Therapeutics* citing dill as a natural remedy for depression.

¾ cup cooked chickpeas, drained and rinsed

2 teaspoons tahini

1 tablespoon fresh lemon juice

2 teaspoons olive oil

1 cup baby spinach leaves

½ cup coconut yogurt

2 tablespoons pine nuts, plus more for topping

2 tablespoons fresh dill leaves

Sea salt and freshly ground black pepper to taste

1 tablespoon chopped fresh dill leaves, for garnish

1. In a food processor, combine the chickpeas, tahini, lemon juice, oil, baby spinach, coconut yogurt, the 2 tablespoons pine nuts, dill leaves, and salt and pepper. Process until smooth.

2. Place the hummus in a serving bowl and sprinkle with the chopped dill, some pine nuts, and pepper. Serve with fresh veggies.

happy cow spinach and artichoke dip

MAKES 1 CUP

Creamy recipes, which often feel comforting, can still be part of your life—even without eating dairy! This version of a classic dip replaces the sour cream, cream cheese, Parmesan cheese, and mayonnaise with cashews and coconut milk to create a still creamy, delectable version that is nourishing and noncongestive.

Dip some veggie sticks in this, and you'll also load up on zinc, magnesium, iron, selenium, and vitamins B_6, E, and K, as well as energizing medium-chain triglyceride (MCT) fats from the coconut.

½ cup raw unsalted cashews

½ cup coconut milk

7 ounces artichoke hearts (half of a commonly sourced can or carton), drained and squeezed of water as much as possible

2 teaspoons fresh lemon juice

½ teaspoon sea salt, plus more as needed

½ teaspoon freshly ground black pepper, plus more as needed

1 cup baby spinach leaves

1. In a blender or food processor, blend the cashews, coconut milk, artichoke hearts, lemon juice, ½ teaspoon sea salt, and ½ teaspoon pepper on high speed until the mixture is very creamy, about 1 minute.

2. Meanwhile, add 2 tablespoons water to a saucepan and heat over medium heat, then add the spinach and cook until the spinach is wilted. Allow it to cool, then squeeze out any excess water. Add the spinach to the blender and blend quickly to break it up, about 5 seconds.

3. Scoop the mixture into the saucepan. Heat it on the stove top over low-medium heat until warmed through, about 5 minutes, stirring frequently. Season with salt and pepper to taste. Serve warm with raw or cooked veggies.

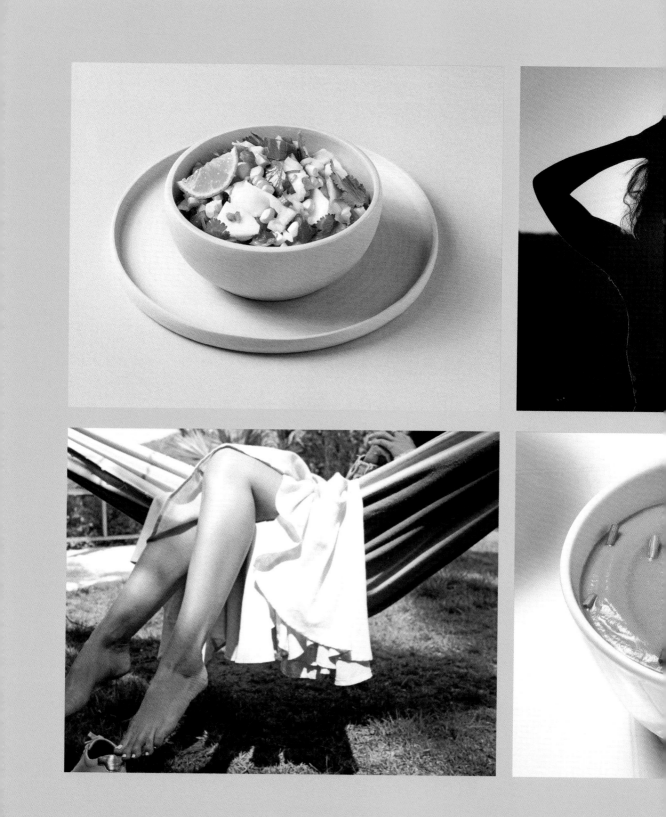

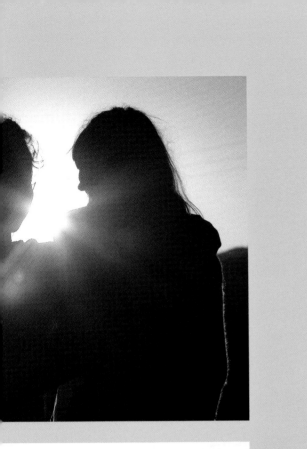

soups and stews

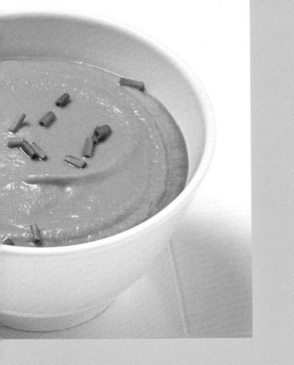

Soups and stews are the ultimate comforting, nourishing food. These dishes are rich in minerals, protein, and fiber. The cooking process partially breaks down the fiber, which makes them easier to digest for those who have difficulty with raw veggies; it can also aid the body's uptake of certain nutrients. Raw and cooked veggies are both important in our diet.

Whether it's cold or hot outside, or it's afternoon, evening, or even late morning, it's always a great time for soup! The variety of nourishing and delicious recipes in this section will cleanse your system and support your beautiful vitality.

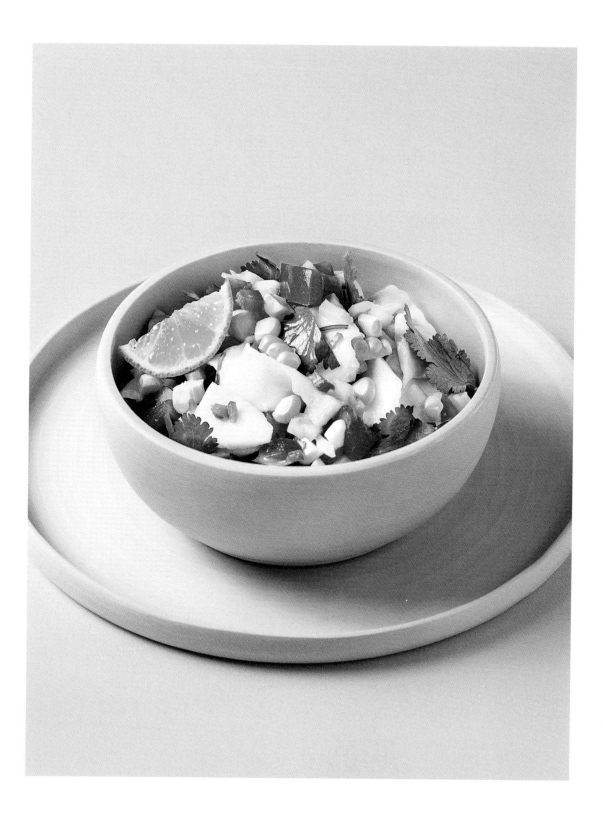

coconut ceviche

SERVES 1 OR 2

Young coconuts from tropical places are an incredible beauty and wellness food, containing medium-chain triglyceride fats that can boost fat burning and provide us with energy, as well as electrolytes like potassium and other minerals. You can source them in health or Asian markets. They are usually shaved down to the white husk interior, with a flat bottom and a pointy cylinder top.

Ceviche is a dish typically made of raw fish marinated in lime or lemon juice and seasonings. For various reasons, not the least of which is that fish is often highly contaminated with heavy metals and other toxins, it is wise to cut out or limit fish consumption. But that doesn't mean we can't enjoy ceviche! Try this version, which is incredibly fresh and tasty, with lime, fresh veggies, herbs, and the satisfying fattiness of the coconut chunks.

Meat from 1 young coconut opened with a large cleaver (see my YouTube video for instructions) and then scraped out with a spoon and cut into 1-inch pieces

1 large Roma tomato, diced

1 cup organic corn kernels, fresh or frozen and thawed

1 cup chopped fresh cilantro leaves

1 red bell pepper, cored, seeded, and diced

¼ cup diced yellow onion, rinsed in cold water and drained

1 teaspoon minced fresh jalapeño

2 tablespoons fresh lime juice (from about 1 medium lime)

2 tablespoons olive oil

½ teaspoon sea salt

In a large bowl, toss all the ingredients together. Cover and refrigerate for at least 1 hour to allow the flavors to meld before serving.

self-love cauliflower soup

SERVES 4

Whenever you need some extra love in a bowl, this is it. It's made of pureed veggies and herbs, gifts straight from nature, and each spoonful supplies you with nourishment, beauty fat, and minerals that give you a loving energy boost whenever you need it.

1 tablespoon coconut oil

½ cup diced yellow onion

1 medium head cauliflower (about 2 pounds), cut into florets, stalk discarded

1½ cups shredded green cabbage

1 tablespoon chopped fresh rosemary leaves

1 tablespoon chopped fresh thyme leaves

1½ cups vegetable broth

1½ cups coconut milk

Sea salt and freshly ground black pepper to taste

1. In a large pot, heat the coconut oil over medium heat. Add the onion, cauliflower, cabbage, rosemary, and thyme, and sauté until the cauliflower starts to slightly brown, about 4 minutes or so. Stir in the vegetable broth and let it simmer, partially covered, for 30 minutes.

2. Transfer the mixture to a blender in batches, taking care with the hot liquid, and blend until smooth. Pour it back into the pot and stir in the coconut milk, warming it to just under a boil. Season with sea salt and pepper.

ginger cabbage cleanse soup

SERVES 6

Feeling heavy, either physically, emotionally, or mentally? Choosing a cleansing meal can help lighten how you feel on any level. And this is a particularly wonderful cleansing recipe, as cabbage is a cruciferous veggie that helps your liver break down toxins so they can be more easily expelled. It is also a natural diuretic with great skin-supporting properties. Ginger boosts our metabolism and can promote better digestion and the expulsion of toxins as well.

Make a full batch for yourself or your household to eat over a few days, if you feel like you need to reset or flush out your system.

1 tablespoon coconut oil

5 cups shredded green cabbage

2 cups diced celery (from 8 celery stalks)

2 cups diced unpeeled zucchini, (from 2 medium zucchini)

2 quarts (64 ounces) vegetable broth

2 bay leaves

1 (1½-inch) piece fresh ginger, peeled and sliced

1½ teaspoons sea salt

1 teaspoon freshly ground black pepper

1. In a large stockpot, melt the coconut oil over medium heat. Add the cabbage, celery, and zucchini, and sauté for about 5 minutes, until softened.

2. Add the vegetable broth, bay leaves, and ginger, and bring to a boil; lower the heat to a simmer and cook, uncovered, for about 15 minutes. Season with the sea salt and pepper.

curried radiance carrot soup

SERVES 4

If we want to be radiant in the world, we have to eat radiant foods! And carrots are one of the best glow-promoting foods around, being high in beta-carotene, which converts to skin-healing vitamin A. This is a delicious soup that includes warming ginger and curry, which possesses anti-inflammatory properties. Serve with some toasty gluten-free bread for a nice contrasting crunchy texture.

1 tablespoon coconut oil, plus more as needed

½ cup chopped yellow onion

8 medium carrots, cut into 3-inch lengths

3 cups vegetable broth

½ teaspoon peeled and grated fresh ginger

1 teaspoon curry powder

½ teaspoon ground turmeric

2 cups coconut milk

Sea salt to taste

1 tablespoon chopped fresh chives

1. In a large saucepan, melt the coconut oil over medium-high heat and sauté the onion for 2 to 3 minutes, until softened.

2. Add the carrots, vegetable broth, ginger, curry, and turmeric, and bring to a boil, then reduce to medium and cook until the carrots are soft, about 15 minutes.

3. Transfer the hot soup to a blender in batches, working carefully with the hot liquid, and blend until smooth.

4. Return the soup to the same pot and heat it back up, adding the coconut milk. Season with sea salt and top with the chopped chives.

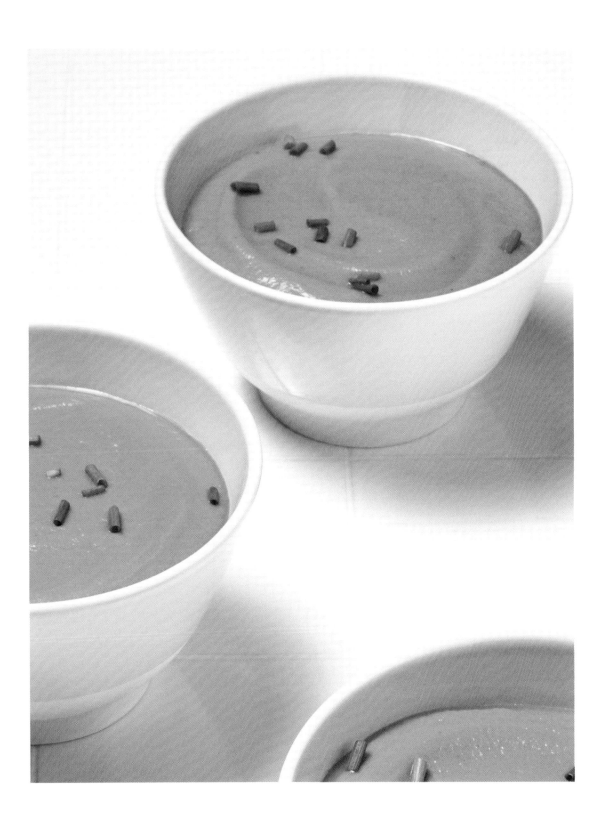

morning miso veggie soup

SERVES 4

I get a lot of questions about what to eat in the morning if you are still hungry after our core morning practice, which includes the Glowing Green Smoothie (aka GGS; page 99). There are many possibilities, including the options presented in the Brunch chapter (see page 213), oatmeal made with water, or a gluten-free avocado and sprout wrap (which I myself eat often). This soup is another great choice for midmorning and beyond. The liquid component is filling, warming, and full of amino acids, beta-carotene, fiber, and other nutrients. It's inspired by the miso soup served at breakfast in Japan, one of my most favorite countries to visit. If you've never tried savory soup in the morning, give it a go, and you might just get hooked!

1 tablespoon coconut oil

2 celery stalks, diced

2 carrots, peeled and diced

1 cup chopped zucchini

1 cup cooked chickpeas, drained and rinsed

2 tablespoons white miso

Sea salt to taste

1. In a saucepan, melt the coconut oil over medium heat. Add the celery and carrots, and cook until they are tender, 6 to 8 minutes.

2. Stir in the zucchini and chickpeas, and cook for about 2 more minutes.

3. Add 4 cups of water. Bring to a boil; reduce the heat and simmer until the vegetables are tender, about 10 minutes. Remove from the heat.

4. In a small bowl, dissolve the miso in 2 tablespoons cool water and stir it into the soup. Season with the salt.

pureed roasted veggie soup

SERVES 2 TO 4

There's something about spooning up all the farm-fresh veggie goodness in this soup that is healing to your spirit.

Raw and cooked veggies are both important for your health. While there is the raw-food camp, which believes that the enzymes in food should be preserved with no heating at all, and the Ayurvedic camp, which believes foods should largely be eaten cooked, my position is that it's beneficial to include *both* raw and cooked veggies on a daily basis. We get lots of raw veggie goodness in our Glowing Green Smoothie (aka GGS; page 99) every day, and soups like this are great for providing cooked veggies. Before eating cooked foods, taking digestive enzymes is recommended to optimize nutrient assimilation. And in the case of tomatoes, the powerful antioxidant lycopene is more easily absorbed when it's cooked.

6 ripe beefsteak tomatoes, halved and cored

2 leeks, trimmed, white and pale green parts cut into ½-inch pieces

2 carrots, cut into ¼-inch pieces

2 tablespoons coconut oil, melted

Sea salt and freshly ground black pepper to taste

3½ cups (28 ounces) vegetable broth

¼ cup chopped fresh basil leaves

1. Preheat the oven to 425°F.

2. In a roasting pan, toss the tomatoes with the leeks, carrots, and coconut oil. Lightly season with sea salt and pepper. Spread the vegetables in a single layer, tomatoes cut sides down, and roast until tender, about 30 minutes. Let them cool down enough to handle, then, using tongs, peel off the tomato skins.

3. In a stockpot, bring the vegetables, broth, and 1 cup of water to a boil. Reduce the heat and simmer, covered, for 10 minutes.

4. Transfer the soup to a blender in batches, working carefully with the hot liquid, and puree. Return the pureed soup to the stockpot, stir in the basil, and adjust the seasonings as desired.

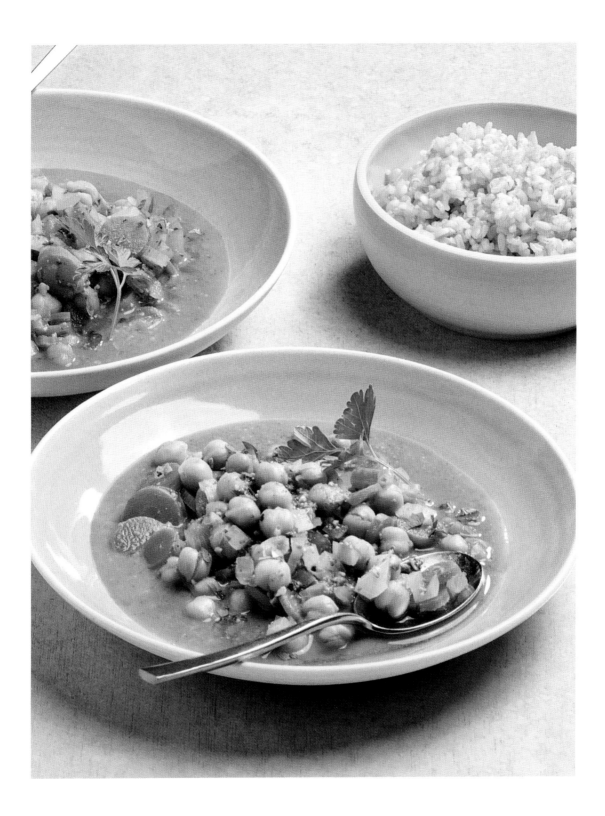

chickpea stew
with pistachio pesto

SERVES 2

Have you ever had pesto in a stew? It's delicious! Pesto, made of freshly ground basil and nuts, is a delicious way to nourish yourself with minerals, antioxidants, and protein. The detoxifying aspect of this recipe comes from omitting the cheese, extra oil, and even the garlic (see page 84), which can be a bit agitating. You will start feeling so amazing as you go along your continuing detox journey toward lightness that you won't even miss those ingredients in this dish. Chickpea Stew is so hearty it makes a fantastic main course. Serve with brown rice (preferably soaked and sprouted).

pistachio pesto

1 cup raw unsalted pistachios

1 cup fresh basil leaves, plus more for garnish

¼ cup olive oil

¾ teaspoon sea salt

1 teaspoon fresh lemon juice

chickpea stew

½ cup diced yellow onion

½ cup sliced carrots

½ cup sliced celery

4 cups (32 ounces) vegetable broth

2 cups cooked chickpeas, drained and rinsed

Sea salt to taste

¼ cup coarsely chopped fresh parsley

1. Make the pistachio pesto: Combine all the pesto ingredients in a food processor or mortar and pestle. Process or mash together, retaining some chunky texture.

2. To make the stew, combine the onion, carrots, celery, and vegetable broth in a large pot and bring to a boil. Lower the heat to a simmer, and cook for about 15 minutes, until the veggies are soft. Add the cooked chickpeas and ½ cup of the pesto, and simmer over low heat for an additional 10 minutes. Season with salt. (Save the rest of the pesto to use as a veggie dip; it will keep for up to 5 days in the refrigerator in an airtight container. We just had to make a larger amount to ensure easier blending.)

3. Ladle the stew into bowls and garnish with the chopped parsley.

nourish stew
with white beans

SERVES 4

This simple stew is surprisingly delicious and strengthening for your body, while being easily digestible. It is high in protein, minerals such as iron, folate, magnesium, and copper, as well as vitamin B_1.

1 tablespoon coconut oil

2 large carrots (about ½ pound total), sliced into ½-inch-thick rounds

3 medium red potatoes (about ½ pound total), cut into ½-inch pieces

½ head cauliflower (about 1 pound), cut into florets

1 medium ripe tomato, cored and chopped

4 cups vegetable broth

2 cups shredded green cabbage (½-inch-wide strips)

2 cups cooked white beans (cannellini or navy), drained and rinsed

1 bay leaf

1 teaspoon Italian seasoning

1 cup baby spinach

Sea salt and freshly ground black pepper to taste

1. In a saucepot, melt the coconut oil over medium heat. Add the carrots, potatoes, cauliflower, and tomato, and sauté for 3 to 4 minutes, until the veggies start to soften.

2. Add the vegetable broth and bring to a boil, then quickly reduce the heat to a simmer. Add the cabbage, white beans, bay leaf, and Italian seasoning, and simmer, covered, for about 20 minutes. Stir in the baby spinach, and season with sea salt and pepper before serving.

asian quinoa soup

SERVES 2

Rice soups are really popular in Asia, and I love having a side of brown rice to eat with my veggie soups. In this variation, we use quinoa instead of rice. It's simple but comforting and a great soup to make on a snuggly evening. Simplifying our foods and our schedules is a great way to help quiet the mind. Feel free to include other veggies as well, adding those that look good at the farmers' market!

1 tablespoon coconut oil

4 green onions (scallions), white and green parts, sliced into ¼-inch pieces

2 teaspoons peeled and grated fresh ginger

1 small fresh red chile, thinly sliced

½ cup quinoa, soaked overnight, rinsed well, and drained

4 cups (32 ounces) vegetable broth

1 tablespoon tamari, plus more to taste

2 cups mixed greens

Freshly ground black pepper to taste

1 large handful cilantro, leaves and stems, coarsely chopped into large sprigs

1. In a large pot, heat the coconut oil over medium heat, add the green onions and ginger, and sauté for 2 to 3 minutes, until the green onions just start to brown lightly. Add the chile and quinoa and cook for 1 more minute.

2. Add the vegetable broth and tamari, and bring to a boil, then lower the heat to a simmer and cook, covered, for about 20 minutes. The quinoa will cook through and the veggies will soften as the soup thickens. Toss in the mixed greens to wilt, season with pepper, and ladle into bowls. Top each serving with some fresh cilantro.

everyday awesome soup

SERVES 6

This is a simple, easy-to-make recipe that has everything it takes to rejuvenate your body and soul, even though it is quite light. It contains some lentils for iron and protein, broccoli and other veggie powerhouses, metabolism-enhancing ginger, B-vitamin-rich nutritional yeast (which adds a creaminess to this soup), tofu for even more protein, and flavorful herbs. Adding the lemon after you take it off the heat adds a fresh brightness.

I eat this all the time, and I love it so much I had to share it with you. Enjoy it!

8 cups filtered water

½ cup red lentils

1 bay leaf

1 (1-inch) piece of fresh ginger, peeled and sliced

2 large carrots (about ½ pound total), sliced

1 small head broccoli (about 1½ pounds), cut into florets

2 celery stalks, sliced

1 cup thinly sliced green cabbage

1 cup zucchini half-moons (zucchini cut in half lengthwise and sliced)

1 cup tofu, cut into 1-inch cubes

1 teaspoon Italian seasoning

1 tablespoon nutritional yeast

Sea salt and freshly ground black pepper to taste

1 cup baby spinach

1 teaspoon fresh lemon juice

1. In a large pot, combine the filtered water, lentils, bay leaf, and ginger. Bring to a boil, then reduce the heat to a simmer and cook until the lentils are soft, about 25 minutes.

2. Add the carrots, broccoli, celery, cabbage, zucchini, and tofu to the mixture, stir, and bring back to a boil. Reduce the heat slightly and cook for 3 to 4 minutes, until the veggies start to soften. Stir in the Italian seasoning and nutritional yeast. Season with sea salt and pepper.

3. Remove from the heat. Stir in the baby spinach and lemon juice. Serve immediately.

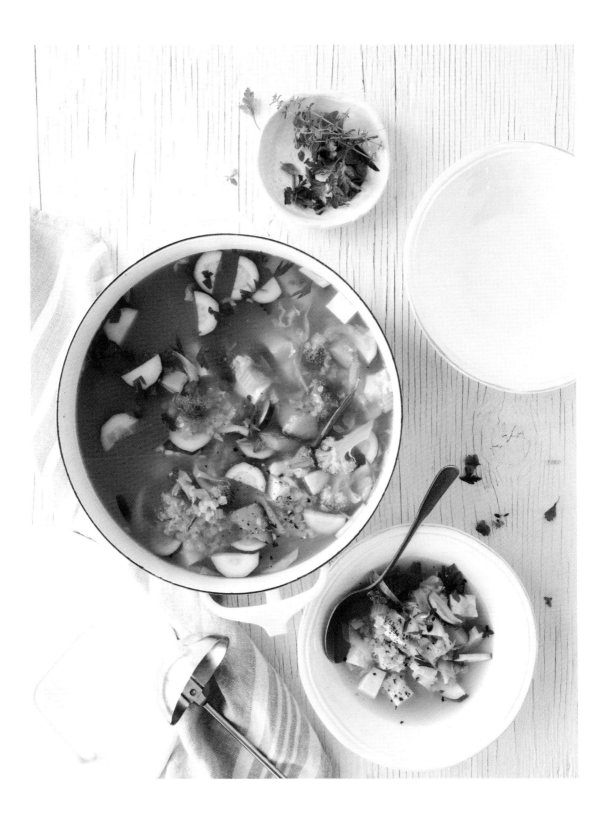

easy miso veggie soup

SERVES 4

Miso is a fermented food that supports healthy digestion. This soup can be made in under ten minutes, so it's perfect for those nights when you just need to throw together a very easy dinner. And I mean easy, as in pour veggie stock into a pot, throw some stuff in, and finish in a few minutes. Doable recipes like this one are important for keeping us properly nourished in our busy lives.

3 tablespoons red miso paste

1 tablespoon tamari

½ teaspoon coconut sugar

6 cups (48 ounces) vegetable stock

2 green onions (scallions), white and green parts, sliced into ¼-inch pieces

1 cup thinly sliced green cabbage

½ cup thinly sliced cremini or shiitake mushrooms

In a large pot, combine all the ingredients. Heat over medium heat (do not let it boil), then reduce the heat and simmer for about 10 minutes. Serve immediately.

pinto bean minestrone

SERVES 4

This version of minestrone is high in protein (from the pinto beans) and has loads of minerals and antioxidants. It doesn't contain pasta, which I don't think it needs as it already contains the beans, or onions and garlic (see page 84). I think you'll be surprised at how delicious this version of minestrone is! Feel free to add other veggies if you want.

2 tablespoons olive oil

2 cups cooked pinto beans, drained and rinsed

1 cup green beans, trimmed and cut on the diagonal into 2-inch pieces

12 cherry tomatoes, halved

1 cup coarsely chopped fresh parsley

6 cups (48 ounces) vegetable stock

Sea salt and freshly ground black pepper to taste

2 cups arugula

¼ cup nutritional yeast

1. In a large stockpot, heat the olive oil over medium heat. Add the pinto beans, green beans, and cherry tomatoes, and cook for 4 minutes or so, until softened.

2. Add the parsley and vegetable stock, and bring to a boil, then reduce the heat to a simmer and cook for about 30 minutes (or a bit less if you don't have the time!). Season with sea salt and pepper.

3. Right before serving, stir in the arugula. Ladle into bowls and sprinkle the nutritional yeast on top.

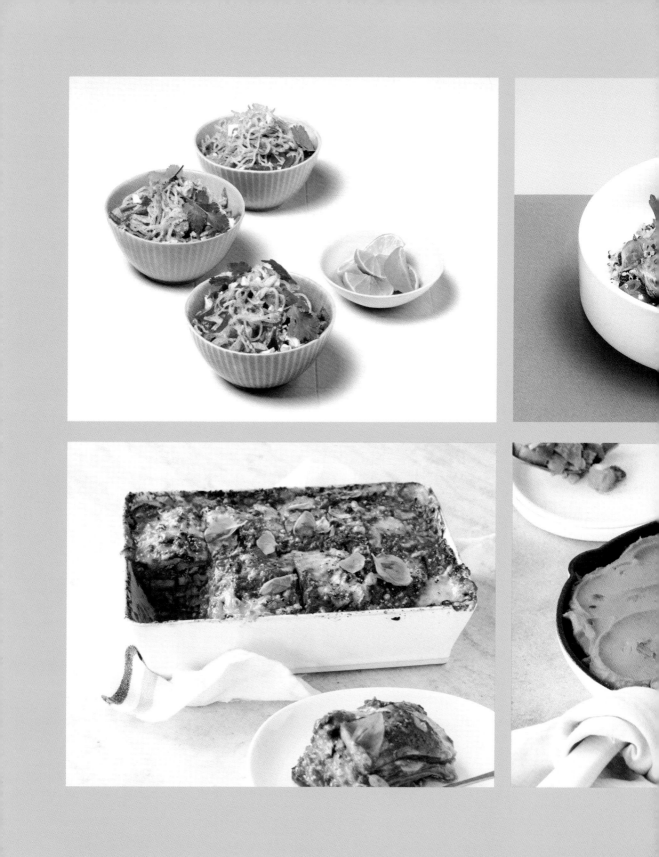

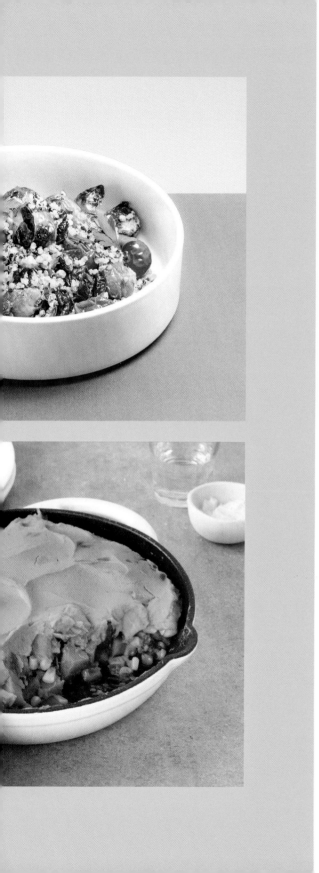

entrées

Clearing out toxins in your body supports you clearing mental blocks, and rejuvenating your body helps you feel more recharged, emotionally and psychologically.

Having tangible tools, such as recipes for your real life, is key to actually putting this information into practice. So here you go! These entrées are all delicious, rejuvenating, and cleansing. You can rotate numerous ones, or just find a few you truly love that call to you, and make them over and over again, rotating the veggies within them.

Like all the other recipes in this book, these are whole-food, plant-based, gluten-free, and properly food combined, so you can experience the power of these principles in your own body and learn to integrate them into your lifestyle long-term.

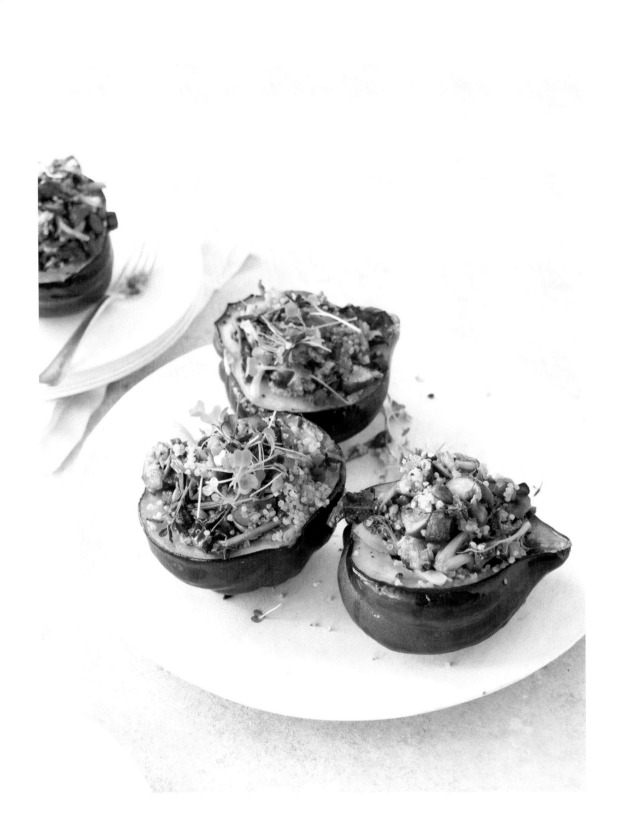

pi stuffed acorn squash

SERVES 4

This yummy recipe is perfect when you want to eat something nourishing with substance to it, yet not feel weighted down. Acorn squash contains vitamin A, niacin, folate, thiamine, and vitamin B_6, and is an especially good source of vitality-enhancing vitamin C.

Squash provides a perfectly imperfect edible bowl from nature to nourish yourself from. Serve with a green salad.

2 medium acorn squash (about 1½ pounds each), halved

1 tablespoon coconut oil, melted

Sea salt and freshly ground black pepper to taste

½ cup quinoa, soaked overnight, rinsed well, and drained

1 tablespoon olive oil

½ cup chopped yellow onion

1½ cups chopped cremini or mixed (cremini, shiitake, portobello) mushrooms

6 ounces (about 3 cups) baby spinach

½ cup coconut milk

1. Preheat the oven to 375°F.

2. Scoop out the seeds from each acorn squash half. Brush the insides with the coconut oil, sprinkle with sea salt and pepper, and bake for 50 minutes, or until soft.

3. In a small saucepan, bring 2 cups of water to a boil and add the quinoa. Bring the water to a simmer, and then lower the heat. Cover and cook for about 14 minutes, until cooked through.

4. While the quinoa is cooking, heat the olive oil in a skillet over medium heat. Add the onion and sauté for 2 to 3 minutes, or until it starts to brown. Add the mushrooms and sauté for 3 to 4 minutes. Add the spinach and season with sea salt and pepper.

5. Combine the cooked quinoa with the onion, spinach, and mushrooms in the skillet. Stir in the coconut milk. Adjust the seasonings to taste.

6. Remove the squash from the oven and stuff the quinoa mixture inside. Place them back in the oven for 8 to 10 minutes, until the stuffing mixture is hot.

gingery basil tempeh and snap peas

SERVES 4

Our minds and bodies are connected. Animal protein is, unfortunately, a primary source of toxicity in the body, not to mention hormones, steroids, and other additives added to the animals' food and environmental toxins absorbed by the animals, including organic and free-range varieties. Therefore, I recommend letting go of animal protein in your diet, or at least scaling way back. Such toxins damage our cells and mitochondria, deplete gluthathione levels, and accelerate aging. Besides protein, this cleansing and rebuilding dish also contains potassium, magnesium, antioxidants, and fiber.

8 ounces tempeh, sliced and then cut into 2-inch pieces

¼ cup tamari

2 tablespoons fresh lemon juice

1 tablespoon plus 2 teaspoons coconut oil

1 (1½-inch) piece of fresh ginger, peeled and grated

1½ cups snap peas, trimmed and "string" removed

½ cup chopped radicchio or red cabbage

1 cup torn fresh basil leaves

Sea salt and freshly ground black pepper to taste

1. Place the tempeh in a single layer in a baking dish. Whisk together the tamari and lemon juice and pour it over the tempeh so it is completely saturated. Cover, refrigerate, and let the tempeh sit in the marinade for at least 20 minutes; in a bind, you don't have to wait as long—just start cooking!

2. In a skillet, melt 1 tablespoon of the coconut oil over medium heat. Drain the marinade from the tempeh, and cook the tempeh for 3 to 4 minutes on each side, until it turns golden brown. Transfer from the skillet to a serving bowl.

3. Turn up the heat slightly, add the remaining 2 teaspoons coconut oil to the same pan, and stir-fry the ginger, snap peas, and radicchio for 3 to 4 minutes, until the veggies are softened yet still crisp. Toss this immediately with the tempeh and the basil. Season with sea salt and pepper, and serve hot!

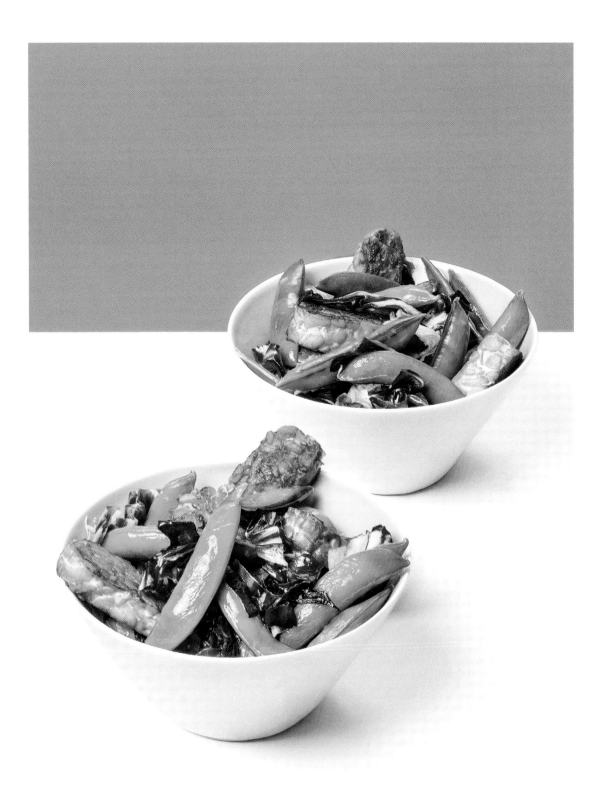

mushroom bolognese

Detoxing is not just about doing a cleanse now and then—although properly administrated cleanses can be enormously helpful. It's about making upgrades, day in and day out, that rejuvenate us and leave us with the experience of feeling good. Soon, though, that experience of feeling amazing will outweigh cravings. Trust me— I've been through it myself in transitioning off cheese, french fries, and pretzels!

In this recipe, chopped mushrooms and veggies replace processed ground red meat. Cremini mushrooms are an excellent source of many minerals, as well as B vitamins and amino acids.

1 tablespoon coconut oil, plus 1 teaspoon if using zucchini noodles

½ cup diced yellow onion

3 cups chopped cremini mushrooms

1 stalk celery, diced

1 carrot, diced

1 (7-ounce) package diced tomatoes, undrained

Sea salt and freshly ground black pepper to taste

2 servings of gluten-free spaghetti , cooked according to package instructions, or zucchini noodles

Splash of olive oil

½ cup torn fresh basil leaves

1. In a large saucepan, melt the 1 tablespoon coconut oil over medium heat, then add the onion, mushrooms, celery, and carrot, and sauté for about 4 minutes, until the veggies soften. Add the diced tomatoes, and cook for about 3 minutes, or until the tomatoes warm and soften into a thick sauce. Season with sea salt and pepper.

2. In a serving bowl, toss the cooked gluten-free spaghetti with the olive oil and a pinch of sea salt. If using the zucchini noodles, melt the 1 teaspoon coconut oil in a saucepan over medium heat, and cook the zucchini noodles for only 2 minutes or so, just to warm them and soften them slightly; transfer the noodles to a serving bowl and add a pinch of sea salt.

3. Serve the veggie mixture on top of the gluten-free pasta or zucchini noodles; garnish with the basil.

one-pot love chili

As your life gets busier, one-pot meals are a lifesaver. They are a practical way to practice self-care by nourishing yourself with low fuss, healthy, delicious meals. This recipe makes a special one-pot meal full of iron and other vitality-supporting minerals, protein for strength and beauty, antioxidants, fiber, and more. Serve with brown rice (preferably soaked and sprouted).

3 tablespoons olive oil

1 medium white onion, diced

1 red bell pepper, cored, seeded, and diced

1½ teaspoons ground cumin

¼ teaspoon cayenne pepper

2 teaspoons chili powder

Sea salt and freshly ground black pepper to taste

2½ cups cooked kidney beans, drained and rinsed

1¾ cups cooked black beans, drained and rinsed

7 cups (56 ounces) diced tomatoes, preferably from cartons or BPA-free cans

1½ cups organic corn kernels, fresh or frozen and thawed

12 ounces organic soy crumbles (optional)

1 avocado, pitted and sliced

1. In a large pot, heat the olive oil over medium heat. Add the onion, bell pepper, cumin, cayenne, and chili powder, and season with sea salt and pepper. Stir together and cook until soft, 3 to 4 minutes.

2. Mix in the beans, tomatoes, and corn. Bring the mixture to a boil, then lower the heat and simmer for 30 minutes, stirring occasionally. Add in the soy crumbles, if desired. Taste and season with sea salt and pepper. Ladle into bowls. Top with the sliced avocado.

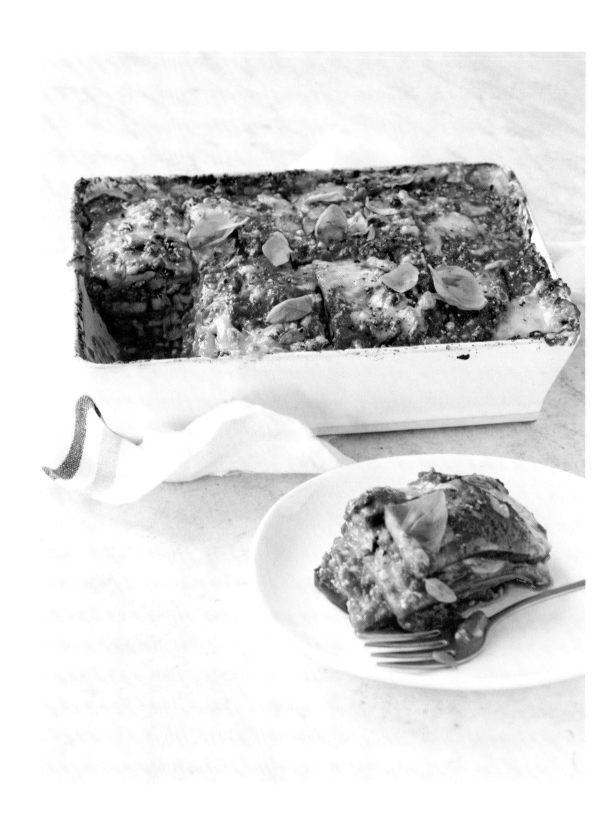

all veggie clean lasagna
with easy red sauce

SERVES 4 TO 6

What we eat translates to our moods, our skin, and how we feel about life. What is amazing about this lasagna is that it's so delicious, you won't even miss the dairy or meat . . . or even the noodles themselves!

easy red sauce

2 tablespoons olive oil

6 ounces tomato paste

25 ounces tomato puree (this is the size for standard packaging; if you find a smaller-size jar or can, go with that and then also add ¼ cup or so of water)

½ cup coarsely chopped fresh basil leaves

Sea salt and freshly ground black pepper to taste

lasagna

Coconut oil

1 large eggplant, peeled and sliced lengthwise into ¼-inch slices (with a mandoline or by hand)

2 zucchini, peeled and sliced lengthwise into ¼-inch slices (with a mandoline or by hand)

4 cups Easy Red Sauce or store-bought red sauce

8 ounces vegan mozzarella cheese

12 ounces crumbled organic, non-GMO tempeh or soy crumbles (optional)

1 cup fresh basil leaves, for garnish

1. Make the easy red sauce: In a medium saucepan, heat the olive oil over medium-low heat; stir in the tomato paste and tomato puree. Reduce the heat to low and cook for about 20 minutes. Stir in the chopped basil and season with sea salt and pepper, then set the pan aside.

2. Preheat the oven to 375°F. Grease a 9 × 9-inch glass baking dish with coconut oil.

3. To make the lasagna, in a skillet, precook the eggplant and zucchini slices in batches, using a small amount of coconut oil for each batch. Cook over medium heat for 1 to 2 minutes on each side.

4. Place a layer of eggplant slices in the prepared glass dish, top it with a layer of zucchini slices, then add a third of the tomato sauce, a third of the vegan cheese, and a third of the crumbled tempeh, if desired. Repeat to make 2 more layers, or until all the veggies are used.

5. Cover the dish with foil and bake for 40 minutes, or until the veggies are softened and the top has browned. Uncover and bake for another 10 minutes. Garnish the top with the basil leaves. Let sit for a few minutes before serving.

mineralizing almond-ginger kelp noodles

SERVES 2

An important way to detox ourselves is through proper mineralization. When we are mineralized, we are balanced and can better fortify ourselves against heavy metals and stress. Sea vegetables, such as kelp, are a great a way to get in a bevy of trace minerals. Kelp noodles, which can be found in the refrigerated section of health markets or sourced online, are virtually calorie-free naturally. Combined with a delicious almond butter, containing vitamin E and protein, and with warming ginger, this is a great nourishing yet cleansing recipe.

sauce

⅓ cup smooth almond butter

2 teaspoons peeled and grated fresh ginger

1 teaspoon sea salt

1 tablespoon maple syrup

1 tablespoon fresh lime juice

1½ tablespoons sesame oil

12 ounces kelp noodles, rinsed with warm water and drained

1 small red bell pepper, cored, seeded, and julienned

1 small carrot, julienned

¼ cup torn fresh basil leaves

¼ cup torn fresh mint leaves

⅓ cup crushed raw unsalted cashews

Handful of fresh cilantro leaves

1. Make the sauce: In a mixing bowl, whisk together all the sauce ingredients. Set to the side.

2. In a large bowl, combine the kelp noodles, bell pepper, and carrot.

3. Pour the sauce over the noodle and vegetable mixture, stir in the basil and mint, and mix evenly. Top with the cashews and cilantro before serving.

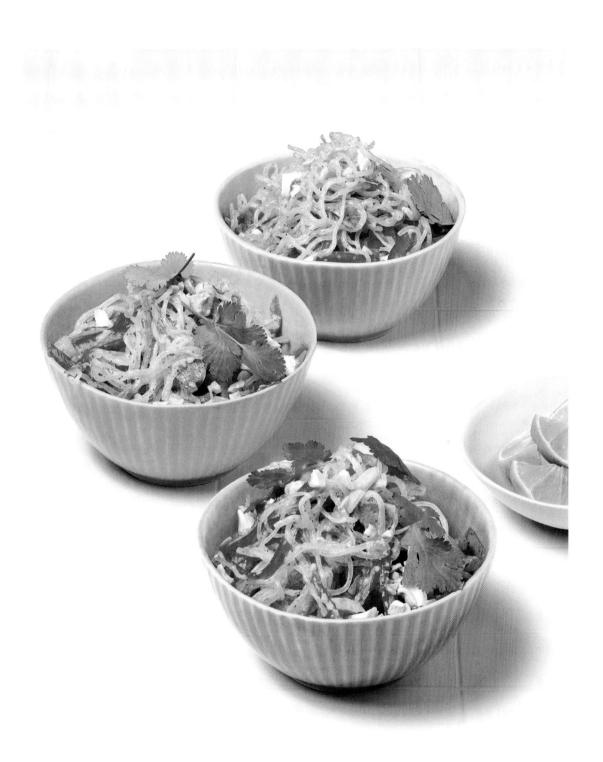

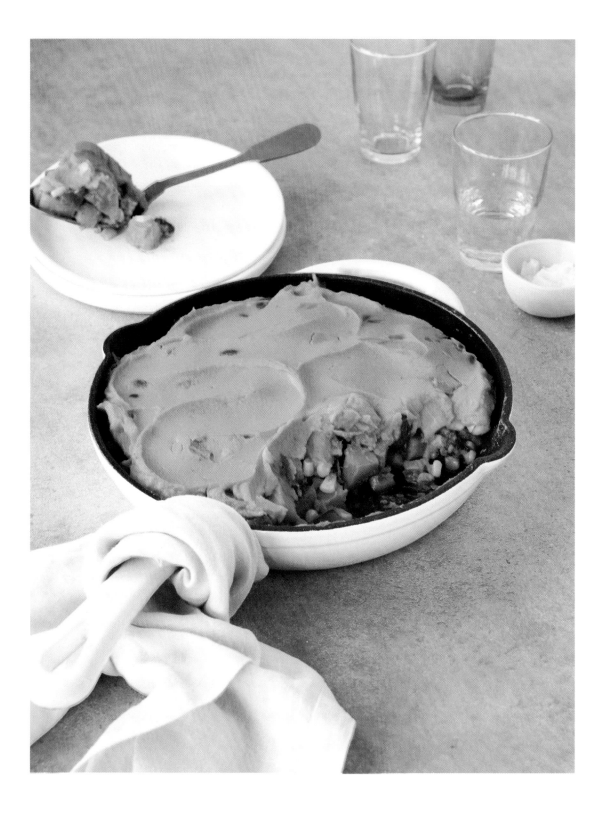

jamaican soul food shepherd's pie

SERVES 6

When you eat this dish, you will be nurturing yourself on a deep level. It's all baked in there—beautiful, vibrant, and nourishing veggies from the earth, protein- and iron-rich kidney beans, and bright herbs and spices. It's inspired by some flavor combinations from the Caribbean. Don't forget to bake in your love!

1 pound sweet potatoes (2 large or 3 medium), peeled

3 tablespoons coconut oil, plus more for greasing

1 yellow onion, diced

1 green bell pepper, cored, seeded, and diced

1 tablespoon peeled and grated fresh ginger

1 large butternut squash (about 3 pounds), peeled, seeded, and cut into 1-inch chunks

1 red habanero pepper, seeded and chopped

2 sprigs fresh thyme

2 bay leaves

Sea salt

½ cup filtered water

1 cup organic corn kernels, fresh or frozen and thawed

1½ cups cooked kidney beans, drained and rinsed

2 teaspoons ground coriander

1 tablespoon ground cumin

1 tablespoon ground mustard

1 tablespoon aniseed

2 tablespoons ground turmeric

2 tablespoons coconut milk

1. Fill a medium pot with water, add the sweet potatoes, and bring to a boil. Reduce the heat slightly and cook until the sweet potatoes are very soft, about 20 minutes. Drain and set aside.

2. In a medium saucepan, melt the 3 tablespoons coconut oil over medium heat, add the onion, bell pepper, and ginger, and sauté for about 3 minutes. Add the butternut squash, habanero, thyme, bay leaves, sea salt to taste, and filtered water. Cover and cook for about 15 minutes, or until the butternut squash is tender. Add the corn, kidney beans, coriander, cumin, mustard, aniseed, and turmeric, and cook for 5 more minutes. Remove the thyme sprigs and bay leaves and discard. Season with sea salt to taste.

3. Preheat the oven to broil.

4. Grease a 9 × 13-inch glass baking dish with coconut oil. Pour the veggie mixture in, spreading it evenly.

5. Place the cooked sweet potatoes in a mixing bowl. Mash with 1 teaspoon sea salt and the coconut milk. Spread the mashed sweet potatoes evenly over the veggie mixture. Broil for about 10 minutes, or until the top browns nicely. Let it sit for at least 10 minutes before serving.

let go gluten-free pasta
with avocado pesto

SERVES 4

Food combining (see page 84 for more info) on a regular basis—as best as you can, in the spirit of perfectly imperfect—is a way to break through to a more cleansed and detoxified body overall, as we continue to make digestion easier and prevent the dreaded bloating!

This recipe is surprisingly delicious and creamy, yet it is gluten-free *and* properly food combined as it contains no nuts. Nuts (protein) are best avoided with pasta (starch), so this avocado pesto is nut-free.

2½ cups fresh basil leaves

2 tablespoons nutritional yeast

1 large avocado, pitted

¼ cup olive oil

¼ teaspoon sea salt

Freshly ground black pepper to taste

1 (12-ounce) package gluten-free pasta, cooked according to package instructions

2 ripe tomatoes, diced

1 tablespoon chopped fresh parsley or chives

1. In a food processor or mortar and pestle, combine the basil, nutritional yeast, avocado, oil, sea salt, and pepper, and process until mixed, retaining some texture.

2. Toss with the freshly cooked (and ideally still warm) pasta and top with the tomatoes and parsley.

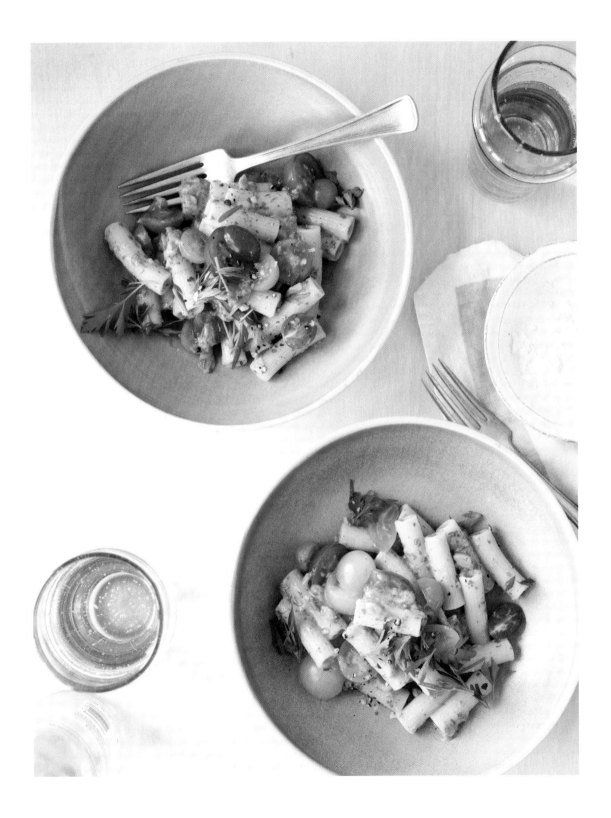

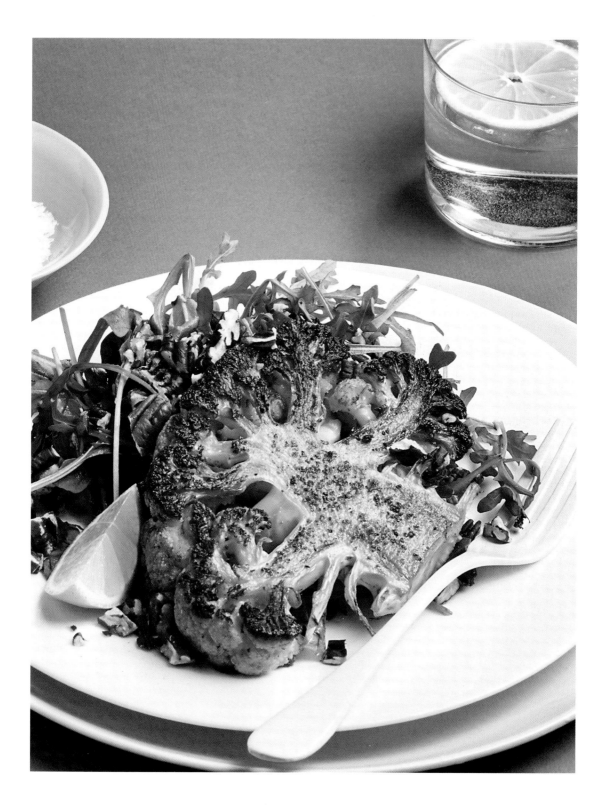

roasted curry cauliflower steak
with wilted greens and pecans

SERVES 4

Eating nourishing veggie-centered entrées is a powerful way to keep your body cleansed on an ongoing basis. And, as our diet becomes lighter, we will have more energy and feel lighter in our minds.

Cauliflower is a great anti-inflammatory, nutrient-rich food. When roasted and served over a salad and pecans, it makes a simple, protein-rich, and satisfying meal that looks beautiful on the plate.

¼ cup coconut oil, melted, plus more for greasing

1 tablespoon curry powder

Freshly ground black pepper to taste

Sea salt

1 large head cauliflower (about 3 pounds), sliced lengthwise through the core into 4 "steaks"

5 ounces (about 5 cups) arugula or mixed salad greens

Squeeze of fresh lemon

½ cup halved or chopped pecans

1. Preheat the oven to 425°F.

2. Whisk together the coconut oil, curry powder, pepper, and a sprinkle of sea salt. Brush both sides of the cauliflower slices with the mixture and place them on a baking sheet. Roast for 25 to 30 minutes, turning them halfway through.

3. Meanwhile, toss the arugula in a bowl with a pinch of sea salt, a squeeze of lemon, and the pecans. Evenly divide the mixture among four plates. Top with the cauliflower steaks.

cumin roasted brussels sprouts
with quinoa

SERVES 4

When we feel good, others can feel it, too, and that is when we are our most beautiful. You know what else makes us feel good? Easy dishes that are tasty, like this one. That is one of the reasons why I love this particular recipe so much.

Brussels sprouts have a surprising amount of protein, and combining them with quinoa creates a complete powerhouse, protein-rich dish. Besides being high in folate (especially important for mamas-to-be), vitamins C and K, potassium, B vitamins, and many other nutrients, Brussels sprouts are excellent for helping to alkalize our bodies and promote good digestion, a key to overall radiance.

2 cups filtered water

1 cup quinoa, soaked overnight, rinsed well, and drained

2 tablespoons coconut oil, melted, plus more for greasing

1 pound Brussels sprouts, trimmed and halved lengthwise

2 cups cherry tomatoes, halved, or 1 Roma tomato, cut into eighths

1 teaspoon ground cumin

Sea salt and freshly ground black pepper to taste

⅓ cup dried cranberries

½ cup chopped fresh parsley or chives

1. In a small pot, heat the filtered water and quinoa over high heat. Once it comes to a boil, quickly reduce the heat to low, cover, and cook for about 16 minutes, until the quinoa is totally cooked through. Fluff with a fork and set to the side.

2. Preheat the oven to 425°F. Grease a 9 × 13-inch glass baking dish with coconut oil.

3. In a bowl, toss the 2 tablespoons coconut oil with the Brussels sprouts and tomatoes. Transfer to the prepared baking dish and roast for about 20 minutes, or until the veggies are softened to your liking.

4. Transfer the veggies to a large serving dish and toss with the quinoa, cumin, sea salt and pepper, and cranberries. Adjust the seasonings as needed. Fold in the chopped parsley.

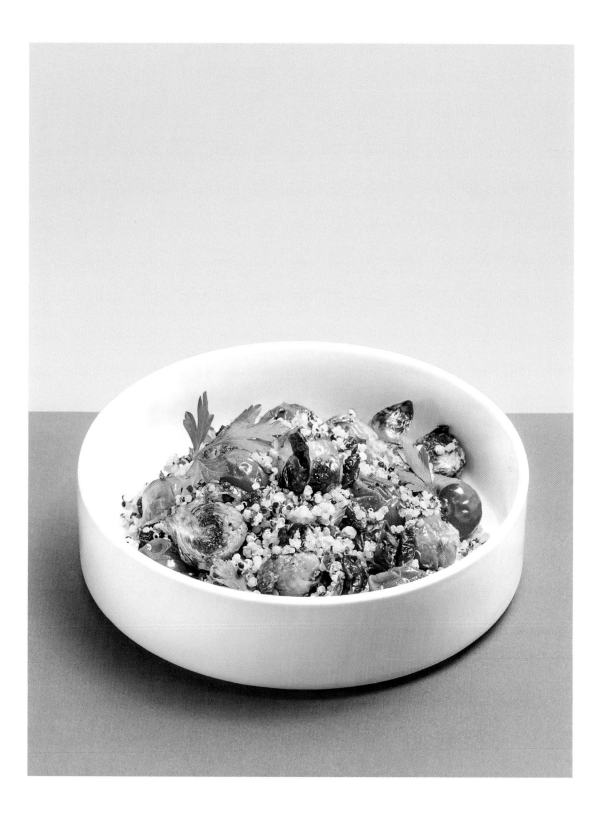

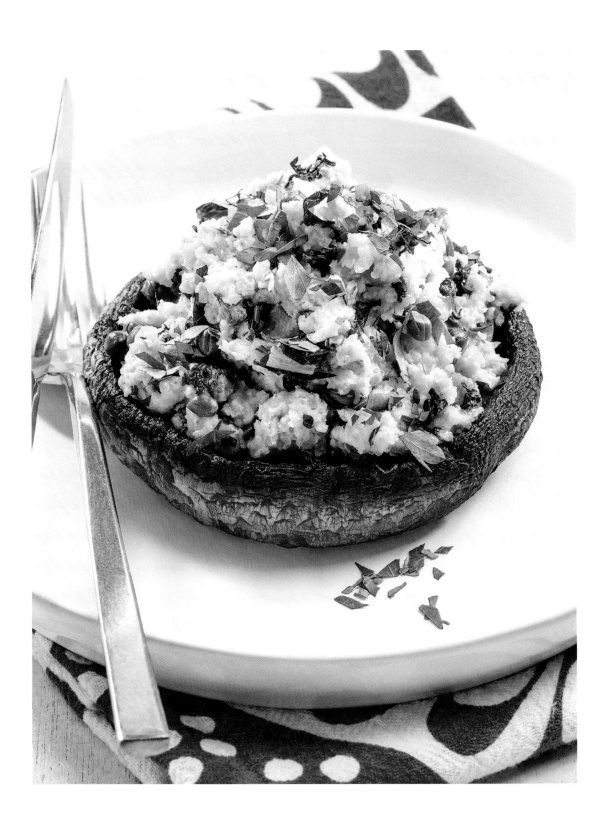

millet magic stuffed 'shrooms!

SERVES 4

Millet is a nutritional staple around the world. In fact, about one-third of the world eats millet as a vital source of nourishment. It's rich in protein and minerals such as magnesium and calcium. Millet makes a hearty stuffing for our portobellos in this recipe, and the pop of rosemary, thyme, and capers adds an interesting flavor combination to revive your senses, in case you've been in a bit of a food—or life—rut.

1 tablespoon coconut oil, plus more for greasing

4 portobello mushrooms, as deep as possible for stuffing

Sea salt and freshly ground black pepper to taste

½ cup millet, rinsed and soaked, preferably overnight

1 medium carrot, diced

½ cup minced kale

2 teaspoons chopped fresh thyme, or ¾ teaspoon dried

2 teaspoons minced fresh rosemary, or ¾ teaspoon dried

⅓ cup drained whole capers

½ cup coconut milk

½ cup coarsely chopped fresh cilantro or parsley leaves, for topping

1. Preheat the oven to 375°F.

2. Grease a baking sheet with coconut oil. Using a spoon, remove the stems and black gills from the portobello mushrooms. Place the portobellos on the prepared baking sheet, cap sides up, and lightly sprinkle with sea salt and pepper. Bake for 20 minutes. Remove from the oven and set to the side.

3. Meanwhile, in a saucepan, bring 2 cups of water to a boil, then quickly reduce to low. Add the millet, cover, and cook for about 20 minutes, until cooked through. Fluff with a fork, drain off any excess water, and set to the side.

4. In a skillet, melt the 1 tablespoon coconut oil. Add the carrot and kale, and cook until softened, about 3 minutes. Stir in the millet, thyme, rosemary, capers, and coconut milk. Season with sea salt.

5. Flip the portobello mushrooms over so they are cap sides down, and stuff the millet mixture into each mushroom's open side. Top with the cilantro before serving immediately.

easy sweet potato
and pinto bean enchiladas

MAKES 8 ENCHILADAS

When we were testing this recipe, the enchiladas kept cracking, so Diego, the manager at our Solluna Juice Bar at the Four Seasons in Beverly Hills, and his family suggested warming the tortillas and soaking them in the salsa before rolling. Bam! Issue fixed. Thank you, Diego, Evelia, and the rest of the fam.

Coconut oil, for greasing

2 medium sweet potatoes (about ½ pound total), peeled

2 large Roma, vine-ripened, or heirloom tomatoes (around 1¾ pounds total)

¼ cup chopped white onion (optional)

2 cups coarsely chopped fresh cilantro leaves

Sea salt to taste

1½ cups coconut milk

2 cups cooked pinto beans, drained and rinsed

8 organic, non-GMO corn tortillas

1 medium avocado, pitted and sliced

1. Preheat the oven to 400°F. Grease a 9 × 13-inch glass baking dish with coconut oil.

2. Fill a pot about halfway with water, add the sweet potatoes, and bring to a boil. Reduce the heat and cook for about 15 minutes, or until tender.

3. Meanwhile, in a blender or food processor, process the tomatoes, onion if desired, ½ cup of the cilantro, and sea salt. Set to the side.

4. Once the sweet potatoes are cool, scoop the flesh into a large bowl, and using a fork, mash them with the coconut milk. Gently stir in the pinto beans. Season with sea salt.

5. Pour the blended tomato mixture into a shallow glass dish. Warm the tortillas in a skillet over low heat and, while still warm, dip each tortilla into the tomato mixture. Spoon one-eighth of the sweet-potato mixture onto the middle of each tortilla, roll them up, and place them side by side, seam-side down, in the prepared baking dish. Bake for about 20 minutes.

6. To serve, place 2 to 4 enchiladas on each plate, and top each portion with some of the remaining tomato mixture, sliced avocado, and cilantro.

jc's lemon fresh green beans
and mushrooms atop quinoa

SERVES 4

When I was backpacking in Thailand, I met a tattooed photographer named JC from the South of France, and we continued to meet periodically in countries like Japan and while I was camping in Africa. JC was a great chef, even using a camping stove! This dish reminds me of the fresh and tasty haricots verts, which are a thinner version of green beans, that he would make. We shared some crazy adventures together, taught each other a lot, and remain friends to this day, and so, Jean-Christophe, this one is in honor of you.

⅔ cup quinoa, rinsed and soaked or sprouted

1 tablespoon coconut oil

4 cups green beans (about ½ pound), trimmed and cut on the diagonal into 2-inch pieces

1 pound cremini mushrooms, thinly sliced

2 tablespoons fresh lemon juice

1½ tablespoons flax oil or olive oil

Sea salt and freshly ground black pepper to taste

⅓ cup pitted and halved black olives

2 tablespoons chopped fresh chives

1. In a saucepan, bring 1⅓ cups of water to a boil, add the quinoa, and quickly reduce the heat to low, cover, and simmer until the quinoa is cooked through, about 16 minutes. When it is done, drain off any excess water and place the quinoa in a serving dish.

2. Meanwhile, in a large skillet, melt the coconut oil over medium-high heat, and sauté the green beans and mushrooms for 3 to 4 minutes, until softened. Turn off the heat and set the pan to the side.

3. In a small bowl, mix the lemon juice, flax oil, sea salt, and pepper, and toss it with the veggies. Arrange the veggies on the quinoa, and top with the halved olives and chopped chives.

twice-baked rosemary, broccoli, and kale–stuffed sweet potatoes

Rosemary contains potent medicinal properties and is a wonderful self-care food to incorporate into your diet. The most interesting health benefits of rosemary include its ability to boost memory, improve mood, reduce inflammation, relieve pain, protect the immune system, stimulate circulation, detoxify the body, protect the body from bacterial infections, prevent premature aging, and heal skin issues.

2 large sweet potatoes (about 1¼ pounds total)

2 teaspoons coconut oil

1 cup very small broccoli florets (no stems)

6 large Tuscan kale leaves, destemmed and finely chopped

1½ teaspoons chopped fresh rosemary

½ cup coconut milk

2 tablespoons nutritional yeast

½ teaspoon sea salt

Freshly ground black pepper to taste

1. Preheat the oven to 425°F.

2. Scrub the sweet potatoes, then poke each several times with a fork, making sure to press well into the flesh.

3. Place the sweet potatoes on a baking sheet and bake for 50 to 60 minutes, until tender. Remove from the oven and let cool. Keep the oven on.

4. Meanwhile, melt the coconut oil in a skillet over medium heat. Add the broccoli and kale and cook for about 3 minutes, until they start to soften.

5. Once the sweet potatoes are cool, slice them lengthwise. Scoop the potato flesh from the inside into a bowl, leaving at least ½ inch of potato flesh to keep the potato skin intact. Mash the potato flesh with the kale, broccoli, rosemary, coconut milk, nutritional yeast, sea salt, and pepper. Stuff the mixture into the potato skins, return them to the baking sheet, and bake for another 10 minutes, or until the tops brown.

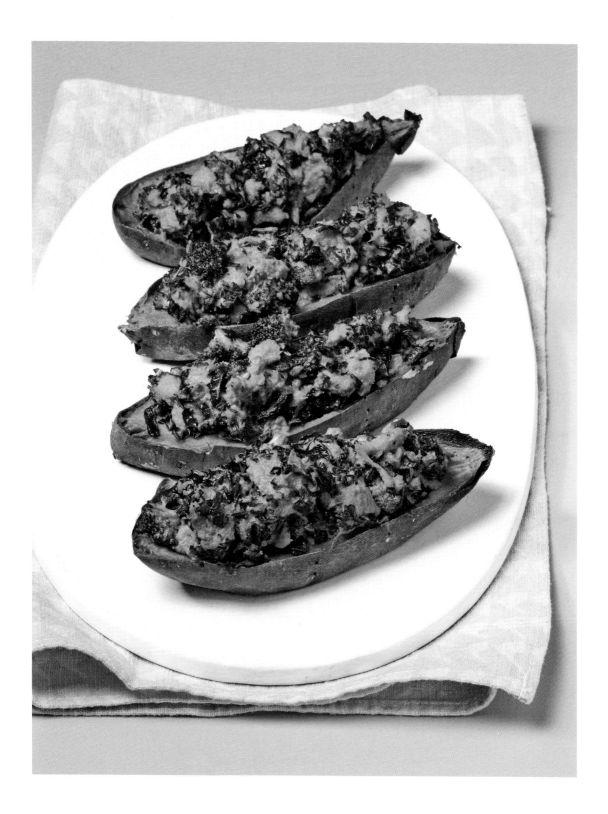

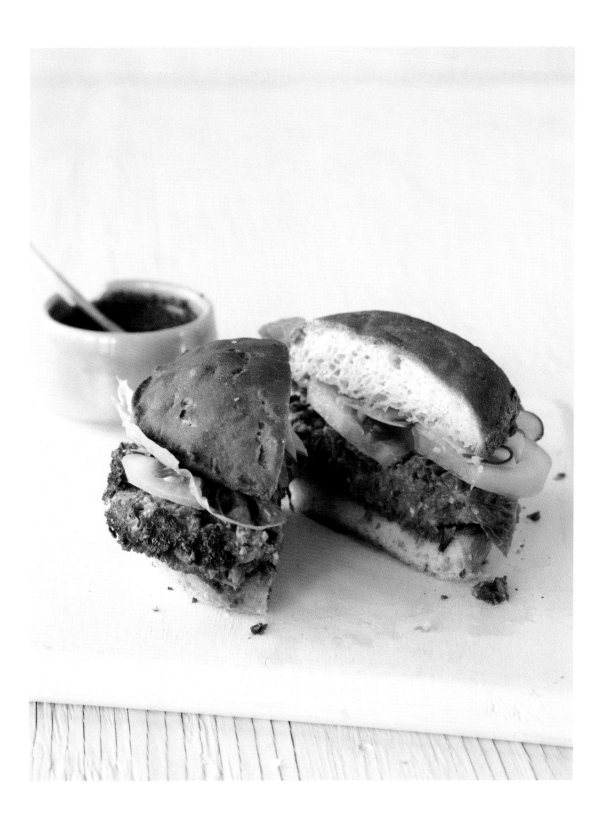

the love thyme veggie burger

MAKES 6 BURGER PATTIES

I love veggie burgers, and I've included one in all of the Beauty Detox books. Here is a simplified version with as few ingredients and as easy to make as possible, in the spirit of food for our real, everyday, crazy lives. Place them on top of salads, tuck them into lettuce wraps, or go for it with some gluten-free bread.

½ cup coarsely chopped yellow onion

1 cup small-diced carrots

12 ounces cremini mushrooms, coarsely chopped

1½ cups cooked and drained green or brown lentils

2 tablespoons coconut oil, plus more as needed

⅓ cup garbanzo bean (chickpea) flour

½ cup minced fresh parsley

1 tablespoon chopped fresh thyme, or 1 teaspoon dried

Sea salt and freshly ground black pepper to taste

Lettuce cups or gluten-free bread

Tomato slices and organic ketchup, for topping (optional)

1. Combine the onion, carrots, mushrooms, and lentils in a food processor and pulse until mixed, but retain some texture. Do not overprocess; otherwise the mixture will become too watery.

2. In a large skillet, melt the 2 tablespoons coconut oil over medium-high heat, and sauté the processed mixture for 3 to 4 minutes, until the veggies soften. Take the pan off the heat and mix in the garbanzo bean flour, parsley, and thyme, and season with sea salt and pepper.

3. Form the mixture into 6 patties about 4 inches across.

4. Using the same pan, heat a thin layer of coconut oil and cook the patties in batches of 3 at time. Cook for 3 to 4 minutes on one side, then flip and cook the other side for 3 to 4 minutes, until cooked all the way through.

5. Serve in lettuce cups or gluten-free bread, and, if desired, top with tomato slices, organic ketchup, and whatever else you like!

lentil love loaf

SERVES 6

Lentils have become a much larger part of my life than even a few years ago. It's partially because of my Ayurvedic studies and partially because Bubby loves them, so they are always around. And now that I routinely eat lentils soaked and sprouted, I don't have bloating or digestive issues from them, so I've fully embraced their amazing health benefits. And on top of all that, they are supereasy to cook and inexpensive.

Lentils are packed with protein and fiber and are naturally low in calories, making them a great food for weight loss. They are also good for energy, can help stabilize blood sugar, and can promote better digestion and cardiovascular health.

This is a hearty dish that is great to serve for dinners and holidays, especially with Ayurvedic-Inspired Mushroom Gravy (page 147) and alongside a salad.

1 cup green or brown lentils

2 cups vegetable broth

1 bay leaf

4 sprigs fresh thyme

1 sprig fresh marjoram

½ teaspoon sea salt

½ teaspoon freshly ground black pepper

2 tablespoons coconut oil

½ cup finely diced yellow onion

½ cup finely diced carrots

½ cup finely diced celery

½ cup finely diced cremini mushrooms

½ cup finely diced broccoli florets

¼ cup thawed frozen peas

1 cup Easy Red Sauce (page 185) or store-bought red sauce

2 tablespoons tamari

1 cup old-fashioned rolled oats

½ cup coconut milk

Ayurvedic-Inspired Mushroom Gravy (page 147)

1. In a small saucepan, combine the lentils, vegetable broth, bay leaf, thyme, marjoram, sea salt, and pepper. Bring to a boil, then lower the heat and simmer, covered, until the lentils are very soft, about 40 minutes. Remove from the heat and allow the lentils to cool. Discard the bay leaf, thyme, and marjoram.

2. Meanwhile, preheat the oven to 350°F. Line the bottom and sides of a 9 × 5-inch loaf pan with parchment paper and set to the side.

3. In a large pot, melt the coconut oil over medium-high heat. Add the onion and sauté until it is soft and translucent, about 5 minutes. Add the carrots, celery, mushrooms, and broccoli, and sauté for 5 more minutes.

4. Add the peas, lentils, red sauce, and tamari to the pot, and continue to sauté until the mixture is heated through, about 2 minutes. Remove from the heat and use a potato masher to coarsely mash the mixture. Keep the majority of lentils and veggies whole; mashing a small amount will simply help bind the loaf.

5. Add the oats and coconut milk to the pot and stir to combine. Pour the mixture into the prepared loaf pan. Use a wooden spoon to spread the lentils evenly and press them down firmly into the edges.

6. Bake for 40 minutes, or until the edges of the loaf are dark brown and beginning to pull away from the sides of the pan. Allow to cool for 10 minutes before removing the loaf from the pan and slicing it. Serve warm, with the mushroom gravy and a salad.

easy protein sage garbanzos

SERVES 2 TO 4

Sage leaf has magical properties. Bundles of it are burned in Native American and other cultures to clear the energy in a space and for special ceremonies. Sage can also be used to help alleviate digestive issues. It has also been associated as a plant medicine that can help ease conditions such as depression and memory loss.

Soaking and sprouting the chickpeas, aka garbanzo beans, yourself is ideal for your digestion. If you buy them precooked, rinse them well and be sure to take two or three digestive enzymes beforehand. If you are interested, you can check out the special digestive enzyme formula on my website. Serve these beans with a big green salad.

1 tablespoon coconut oil

2 cups cooked chickpeas, drained and rinsed

1½ cups chopped lacinato kale

1½ tablespoons minced fresh sage

5 radishes, thinly sliced

1½ tablespoons fresh lemon juice

1 tablespoon olive oil

¼ cup minced fresh parsley

Sea salt and freshly ground black pepper to taste

1. In a saucepan, melt the coconut oil over medium heat, and add the chickpeas, kale, and sage. Cook for 3 to 4 minutes, or until the chickpeas start to brown slightly and the kale softens.

2. Turn off the heat and toss in the radishes, lemon juice, olive oil, and parsley. Season with sea salt and pepper.

lentil tacos

SERVES 4

This dish is pretty delicious, I have to say. The lentils are rich in protein and minerals, and, with a similar consistency, they make a great ground beef replacement.

Plant foods provide all the protein you need, plus some minerals, fiber, and micronutrients that are missing in animal products. Unfortunately, animal agriculture is one of the most destructive industries for Mother Earth, contributing to worldwide deforestation and species extinction, and many other harms (a great documentary to watch about this is *Cowspiracy: The Sustainability Secret*). This is a happy and loving recipe for you, me, and the entire planet!

2 tablespoons coconut oil

2 medium tomatoes, cored and diced

1 cup chopped carrots

2 cups cooked green lentils

½ teaspoon freshly ground black pepper

⅛ teaspoon cayenne pepper

½ teaspoon ground cumin

½ teaspoon ground coriander

1 cup finely chopped spinach leaves

½ cup chopped fresh cilantro leaves

1 cup organic corn kernels, fresh or frozen and thawed

Sea salt to taste

1. In a saucepan, melt the coconut oil over medium heat, add the tomatoes and carrots, and cook for a few moments, until they soften. Add the lentils, black pepper, cayenne, cumin, and coriander, and stir until everything is mixed evenly.

2. Turn off the heat and mix in the spinach, cilantro, and corn. Season with sea salt.

fresh-thyme farinata

SERVES 4

I was eating at an Italian restaurant in Chicago called Spiaggia, and I told the chef I ate plant based. He served a version of this delicious *farinata*, which is a delicious chickpea pancake. It was one of the most creative things I've been served at a nonveg restaurant, and I loved it with the greens they served alongside. Full of protein and minerals, it was a filling entrée, a hearty and rejuvenating dish for sure. Here is a fresh, delicious version you can make for yourself, your friends, or your family.

farinata

2 cups filtered water

½ cup garbanzo bean (chickpea) flour

½ teaspoon sea salt

3 tablespoons olive oil

1 tablespoon chopped fresh thyme

2 teaspoons chopped fresh oregano

1 tablespoon coconut oil, plus more as needed

topping

2 teaspoons fresh lemon juice

1 tablespoon olive oil

Pinch of sea salt

Freshly ground black pepper to taste

5 ounces arugula (about 5 cups)

1. Make the farinata batter: In a bowl, whisk together the filtered water and garbanzo bean flour until smooth. Whisk in the sea salt, olive oil, thyme, and oregano.

2. In a large saucepan, melt the 1 tablespoon coconut oil over medium heat, and pour about a quarter of the batter into the saucepan, making a 6-inch round. Cook for 3 to 4 minutes on one side, until it browns, and then flip and cook the other side for another 3 minutes, or until cooked through as well. Repeat with the remaining batter, adding more coconut oil to the pan if necessary.

3. Prepare the topping: In a large bowl, whisk together the lemon juice, olive oil, sea salt, and pepper, and toss in the arugula.

4. Top the farinatas with the arugula before serving.

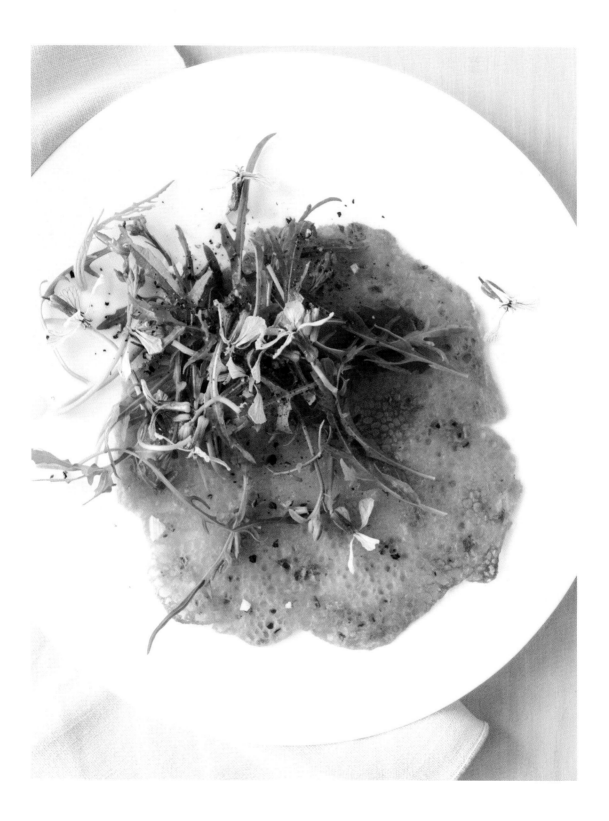

note:
You can purchase sprouted brown rice at the health market, either in the bins or in containers, for a bit higher price. I find it totally worth it, as it makes prep much quicker. It also means you can always have sprouted rice, which is easier for your body to digest and utilize the minerals and nutrition.

vegan party paella

SERVES 6

There is a paella recipe in *The Beauty Detox Foods*, but I was inspired to make a different version after tasting the veggie paella that was served at my friend Jen's birthday party. This is a great dish to serve at parties, or for the everyday party that is your home life, since you'll get good leftover mileage.

2 tablespoons coconut oil, plus more for greasing

3 cups vegetable broth

1½ cups brown rice, rinsed and preferably soaked and sprouted (see Note)

2 red bell peppers, cored, seeded, and cut into 1-inch squares

1½ cups broccoli florets

½ pound asparagus (7 to 9 spears), trimmed and cut on the diagonal into 1-inch lengths

1 zucchini, sliced crosswise and cut into half-moons

1 medium white onion, coarsely chopped

2 large tomatoes, preferably Roma

¾ teaspoon saffron threads

Sea salt to taste

1. Generously grease a 9 × 13-inch glass baking dish with coconut oil.

2. In a saucepan, bring the vegetable broth and the rice to a boil over medium-high heat, then quickly reduce the heat to a simmer, cover, and simmer until the rice is cooked through, about 50 minutes. Set to the side.

3. Meanwhile, in a large skillet, melt the 2 tablespoons coconut oil, add the bell peppers, broccoli, asparagus, and zucchini, and sauté until lightly softened. Set to the side.

4. In a blender, combine 1 cup of water, the onion, and tomatoes. Blend until mixed evenly to the thickness of a consommé.

5. In a large bowl, mix the rice and sautéed veggies, and stir in the consommé. Mix in the saffron and season with sea salt.

6. Preheat the oven to 400°F. Pour the mixture into the prepared baking dish, spreading it into an even layer. Bake until it is hot and the top is browned, about 20 minutes.

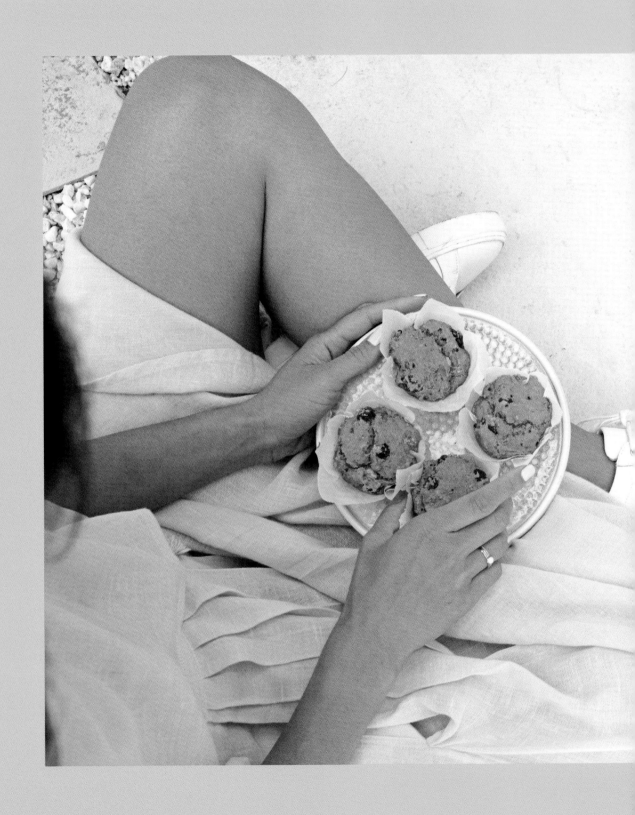

brunch

I'm a big advocate of practicing our incredible morning practice, outlined on page 25, which includes sipping hot water with lemon, taking SBO probiotics, having some meditation or stillness, and drinking the Glowing Green Smoothie. Yet afterward, I totally get that the relaxed, late-morning/early-afternoon weekend ritual of brunch, whether by yourself or with friends and family, can be a fun and soul-nourishing practice. Hence, I want to supply you with some rejuvenating brunch options that are delicious yet won't weight down your energy for the rest of the day!

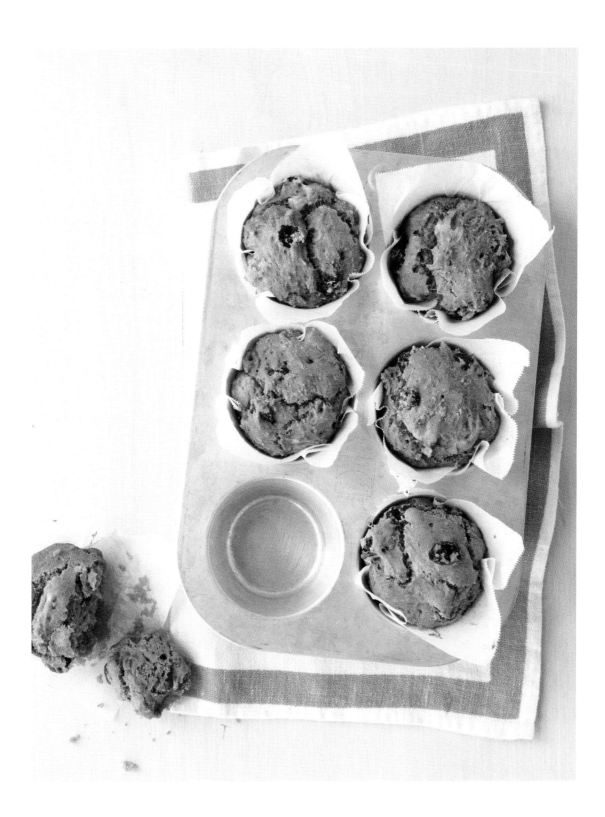

cranberry cinnamon muffins

MAKES 12 MUFFINS

Who doesn't like muffins? The issue is that "regular" muffins often contain ingredients like white flour, vegetable oil, and dairy that can block our guts and, accordingly, our moods and the clarity of our minds. So I created these amazing muffins, which are a huge hit whenever I make them—even with people who are self-proclaimed "not healthy."

It took me a bit of work to get these right; no one said vegan, gluten-free, and properly food combined baking is easy! I am honored and thrilled to offer these delicious muffins to you now, after much trial and error. I hope you love them, too!

2 cups KS Gluten-Free Flour Mix (page 252)

2 teaspoons baking powder

1 teaspoon baking soda

½ teaspoon guar gum

¼ teaspoon sea salt

1 teaspoon ground cinnamon

¼ cup coconut oil, melted

¼ cup coconut nectar

½ teaspoon ground turmeric

½ teaspoon stevia powder

½ cup mashed banana

¾ cup almond milk

¾ cup dried cranberries

1. Preheat the oven to 350°F. Line a muffin tin with 12 paper baking cups.

2. In a large bowl, whisk together the flour mix, baking powder, baking soda, guar gum, sea salt, and cinnamon. Make a well in the middle.

3. Add the coconut oil, coconut nectar, turmeric, and stevia to the well in the bowl, and stir to combine. Add the mashed banana and almond milk, and stir until the liquid is absorbed and the batter is smooth. Stir in the cranberries until evenly distributed.

4. Spoon the batter evenly into the paper cups, filling each about three-fourths full.

5. Bake the muffins for 18 to 20 minutes, or until they are a light golden brown and the tops bounce back when lightly touched with a finger. Let cool for at least 10 minutes on a rack before serving.

pumpkin pie muffins

MAKES 12 MUFFINS

Sharing and connecting with others is part of our true nature, and a great way to do that is with these yummy pumpkin-y muffins, which are easy for everyone to enjoy when served at family brunches, or at midday picnics or get-togethers.

2 cups KS Gluten-Free Flour Mix (page 252)

2 tablespoons pumpkin pie spice

2 teaspoons baking powder

1 teaspoon baking soda

½ teaspoon guar gum

½ cup coconut sugar

¼ teaspoon sea salt

¼ cup coconut oil, melted

¼ cup coconut nectar

1 cup pumpkin puree

¾ cup almond milk

1. Preheat the oven to 350°F. Line a muffin tin with 12 paper baking cups.

2. In a large bowl, whisk together the flour mix, pumpkin pie spice, baking powder, baking soda, guar gum, coconut sugar, and sea salt. Make a well in the middle.

3. Add the coconut oil and coconut nectar to the well in the bowl, and stir to combine. Add the pumpkin puree and almond milk, and stir until the liquid is absorbed and the batter is smooth.

4. Spoon the batter evenly into the paper cups, filling each about three-fourths full.

5. Bake the muffins for 16 to 18 minutes, until they are a light golden brown and the tops bounce back when lightly touched with a finger. Let sit for at least 10 minutes on a rack before serving.

veggie millet hash browns
with radiance carrot ketchup

MAKES 6 TO 8 HASH BROWN PATTIES

This recipe provides a texture and taste similar to good ole hash browns. Yet we are using millet, a restorative food that is extremely nutritious. Though it is technically a seed, we treat it like a grain. It is gluten-free and packed with B vitamins, minerals such as calcium and magnesium, antioxidants, fiber, and protein.

This great variation on hash browns is one way to get some millet into your diet. And for a twist on an organic ketchup sans high fructose corn syrup, check out this tasty carrot ketchup version to top it all off.

radiance carrot ketchup

3 carrots, peeled and cut into 2-inch pieces

2 small beets, peeled and cut into 2-inch pieces

2 tablespoons apple juice

3 tablespoons maple syrup

1 tablespoon raw apple cider vinegar

¼ teaspoon onion powder

¼ teaspoon sea salt, or to taste

hash browns

1 cup millet, soaked overnight, rinsed, and drained well

2 teaspoons coconut oil, plus more as needed

¼ cup diced yellow onion

1 cup chopped cauliflower

½ cup chopped broccoli

½ cup finely chopped carrots

2 tablespoons garbanzo bean (chickpea) flour

½ cup minced fresh parsley

Sea salt and freshly ground black pepper to taste

(RECIPE CONTINUES)

1. Make the carrot ketchup: Place a steamer basket in the bottom of a large stockpot, and add water to reach just below the basket. Place the carrots and beet pieces in the basket, then bring the water to a boil. Reduce the heat to medium-low, cover, and simmer for 10 to 15 minutes, until the carrots and beets are soft.

2. Put the carrots and beets in a blender and add the apple juice, maple syrup, cider vinegar, onion powder, and sea salt. Process until smooth.

3. Transfer the mixture to a small saucepan and bring to a boil, then simmer over medium-low heat for 20 minutes. Cover and refrigerate while making the hash brown patties.

4. Make the hash browns: In a medium saucepan, bring the millet and 3 cups of water to a boil, then reduce the heat to a simmer and cook until the millet is cooked through, 20 to 25 minutes. Drain off any remaining water and set to the side.

5. In a skillet, melt the 2 teaspoons coconut oil over medium heat, add the onion, cauliflower, broccoli, and carrots, and cook until softened, about 5 minutes.

6. In a mixing bowl, mash the veggies and the millet together with a potato masher. Toss in the garbanzo bean flour and parsley and mix well. Season with sea salt and pepper. Let the patties cool so you can handle them (but above room temperature; otherwise, they won't form patties easily), and form 6 to 8 round or oval croquette patties.

7. In the same skillet you used for the vegetables, melt additional coconut oil in a thin layer over medium heat. Add the patties and cook for 3 to 4 minutes on each side, until they turn a nice golden color. Serve with the carrot ketchup.

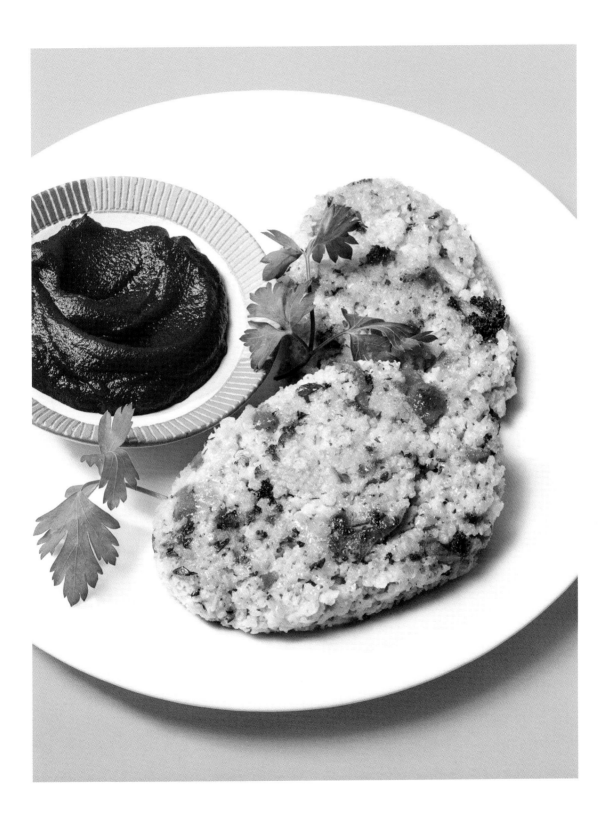

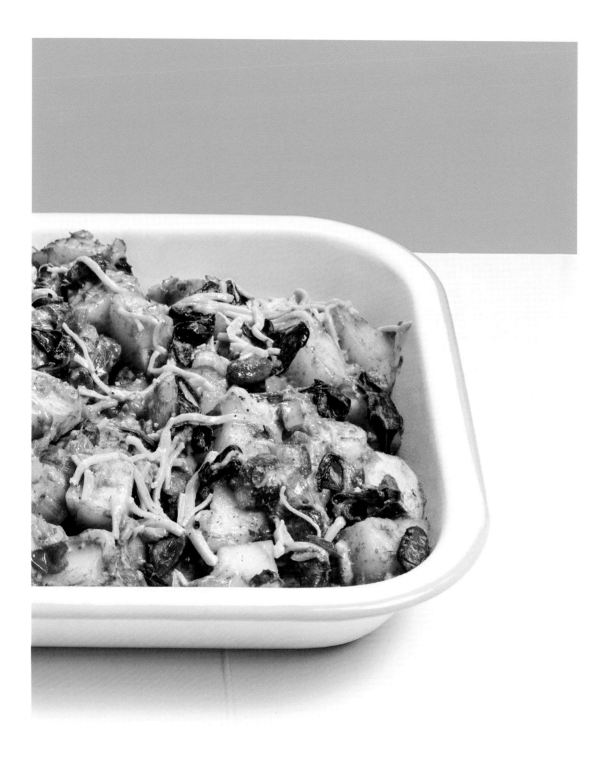

sunday brunch casserole

SERVES 6

This is a warming, flavorful, and soul-nourishing dish. It is so delicious and easy on your digestion (including with vegan cheese, which is pretty tasty these days, swapping out dairy cheese), it might just encourage you to start hosting brunch more often—or maybe just making it more often for yourself!

5 medium russet or long white potatoes (about 1½ pounds total), unpeeled

1 tablespoon coconut oil, plus more for greasing

1 yellow onion, chopped

1 cup diced fresh tomato

2 cups cooked pinto beans, drained and rinsed

3 cups baby spinach

1 teaspoon sea salt, or to taste

Freshly ground black pepper to taste

2 teaspoons smoked paprika

1 teaspoon ground turmeric

1½ cups vegan Cheddar cheese shreds

2 tablespoons garbanzo bean (chickpea) flour

1. In a large saucepan of water, boil the potatoes for about 30 minutes, until they're tender. Drain, peel, and cut them into small cubes; set to the side.

2. Preheat the oven to 350°F. Grease a casserole dish with coconut oil.

3. In a skillet, melt the 1 tablespoon coconut oil over medium heat and add the onion, cooking for 1 minute. Add the tomato, pinto beans, and spinach. Stir in the salt, pepper, paprika, turmeric, and 1 cup of the vegan cheese. Gently stir in the potato cubes and the garbanzo bean flour, then pour the mixture into the prepared casserole dish. Sprinkle the top with the remaining ½ cup vegan cheese and bake for about 20 minutes, or until the top is lightly browned and the vegan cheese has melted.

veggie mini frittatas

MAKES 14 FRITTATAS (ABOUT 2 INCHES IN DIAMETER)

These savory little frittatas are a healthful, rejuvenating brunch food. They kinda look like little muffins yet offer a bevy of nutritious, antioxidant-rich veggies, and protein and B vitamins from the garbanzo bean flour and nutritional yeast.

2 tablespoons coconut oil, melted, plus more for greasing

2 cups garbanzo bean (chickpea) flour

¼ cup nutritional yeast

1 teaspoon baking powder

2 teaspoons chopped fresh rosemary, or ¾ teaspoon dried

1 tablespoon chopped fresh thyme, or 1 teaspoon dried

1 tablespoon chopped fresh oregano, or 1 teaspoon dried

1½ teaspoons sea salt

½ teaspoon freshly ground black pepper

2½ cups coconut milk

3 cups assorted chopped veggies: broccoli, bell pepper, zucchini, carrot, spinach

Miso Mustard Sauce (page 146)

1. Preheat the oven to 400°F. Brush some coconut oil over the cups of a mini muffin tin.

2. In a bowl, combine the garbanzo bean flour, nutritional yeast, baking powder, herbs, sea salt, and pepper with the coconut milk. Whisk until smooth.

3. In a skillet, heat the 2 tablespoons coconut oil over medium heat, add the chopped veggies, and cook until they soften, about 5 minutes. Set to the side to cool.

4. Spoon about 1 tablespoon of the veggie mixture into each of the prepared muffin cups. Add ¼ cup of the garbanzo bean batter to each cup. Stir each muffin cup to make sure the batter gets to the bottom and the veggies are evenly distributed.

5. Bake for 30 to 35 minutes, until a toothpick inserted in the center comes out clean and the frittatas begin to brown on top. Remove and let cool for at least 10 minutes before transferring them to a cooling rack.

smoky tempeh bacon

SERVES 4

This tempeh recipe creates a bacon-like texture that is salty and smoky, with some sweet and acidic flavors.

Okay, it is not *exactly* like regular bacon, but the benefits of having something pretty tasty that also supplies loads of protein and B vitamins, combined with not eating regular bacon—which is a processed meat that contains nitrates, which have been linked to cancer—cannot be overstated. According to the American Institute for Cancer Research, no amount of processed meat is considered safe for consumption. Most foods are okay to eat here and there, but bacon's toxicity puts it in a category to give up altogether, albeit in our personal, perfectly imperfect timing of phasing it out. Enjoy this tempeh bacon with a green salad and veggies.

2 tablespoons tamari

1 tablespoon raw apple cider vinegar

1 tablespoon maple syrup

2 tablespoons olive oil

1 teaspoon smoked paprika

1 teaspoon Dijon mustard

8 ounces tempeh, cut into ¼-inch-thick strips

1. In a small bowl, whisk together all the ingredients except the tempeh.

2. Place the tempeh strips in a single layer in a flat-bottomed casserole dish, and pour the marinade over the top, flipping the tempeh over so that all sides are saturated with the marinade. Cover and let sit for at least 20 minutes at room temperature.

3. Meanwhile, preheat the oven to 350°F.

4. Bake the tempeh with the marinade for 15 minutes, then flip it and bake for another 15 minutes, or until it browns nicely.

happy earth scramble

SERVES 4

This joyful tofu-based scramble is high in protein and B vitamins supplied from the nutritional yeast, and minerals and vitamin D from the mushrooms.

It is also exactly in keeping with the Harvard School of Public Health's recommendation: "Keeping intake of eggs moderate to low will be best for most, emphasizing plant-based protein options when possible." Now that is a happy scramble for your body and whole being!

2 tablespoons nutritional yeast

1 teaspoon chili powder

1 teaspoon ground cumin

¾ teaspoon ground turmeric

1 teaspoon sea salt

2 tablespoons coconut oil

1½ cups sliced cremini mushrooms

1 red bell pepper, cored, seeded, and cut into ½-inch dice

24 ounces organic, non-GMO firm tofu, coarsely chopped

Freshly ground black pepper to taste

1. In a bowl, combine the nutritional yeast, chili powder, cumin, turmeric, and sea salt. Set this spice mix to the side.

2. In a large skillet, melt the coconut oil over medium-high heat. Add the mushrooms and bell pepper, and sauté for 5 to 6 minutes, until everything just starts to brown.

3. Stir in the spice mix and the tofu. Smash the tofu with a spatula to crumble it into a scrambled egg–like consistency. Cook for another 3 to 4 minutes, or until the tofu is thoroughly warmed. Season with pepper before serving.

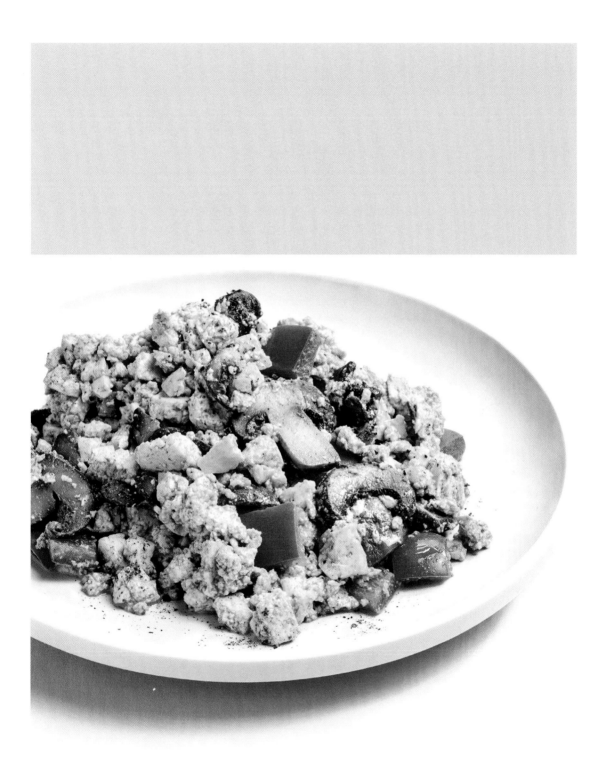

irish corned beef-free and hash

SERVES 4 TO 6

This is a delicious, nourishing version of hash that contains the traditional cabbage and pieces of red bell pepper that emulate the reddish pops of color from the beef in the original recipe. This dish is rich in vitamins A and C, B vitamins, minerals like manganese and copper, and fiber. Foods can open us up and cleanse us. How beautiful is that?

2 tablespoons coconut oil

½ cup chopped yellow onion

2 large sweet potatoes, diced (about 1 pound total)

1 large head green cabbage, shredded (you should have 3 cups)

1 red bell pepper, cored, seeded, and diced

2 tablespoons chopped fresh parsley

Sea salt and freshly ground black pepper to taste

1. In a large skillet, melt the coconut oil over medium heat. Add the onion and sauté for 2 to 3 minutes, until softened. Add the sweet potatoes, cover, and reduce the heat to low. Continue cooking for about 12 minutes, until tender, stirring partway through. When done, stir in the cabbage and bell pepper and cook for 2 to 3 minutes, until softened.

2. Remove the skillet from the heat and stir in the parsley. Season with sea salt and pepper.

eggless ayurvedic frittata

SERVES 2

This is akin to a savory pancake. I first got hooked on it when I made a version of this recipe in an Ayurvedic nutrition class that was part of my Ayurvedic program. Because so many of us adore pancakes, I wanted to include one! The garbanzo bean (or chickpea) flour, also high in protein and iron, is great for binding, eliminating the need for an egg replacer. With no gluten or egg or any animal products, this is as cleansing and digestion-friendly as you can get for any sort of "pancake." Enjoy with a fresh green salad.

½ cup garbanzo bean (chickpea) flour

½ medium sweet yellow onion, diced

½ cup chopped fresh cilantro leaves and stems

½ teaspoon sea salt

1 teaspoon cumin seeds

1 tablespoon coconut oil

1. In a medium bowl, combine the garbanzo bean flour, onion, cilantro, sea salt, and cumin seeds. Mix in ½ cup of water until the mixture is thoroughly combined, though slightly lumpy.

2. In a skillet, melt the coconut oil over medium heat, and using a spatula, pour the batter into the pan. Move the pan around so the mixture spreads into an even flat shape.

3. Cook for 3 to 4 minutes on the first side, and then flip it carefully. It helps to use two spatulas to do this, or cut it into pieces and flip them one by one.

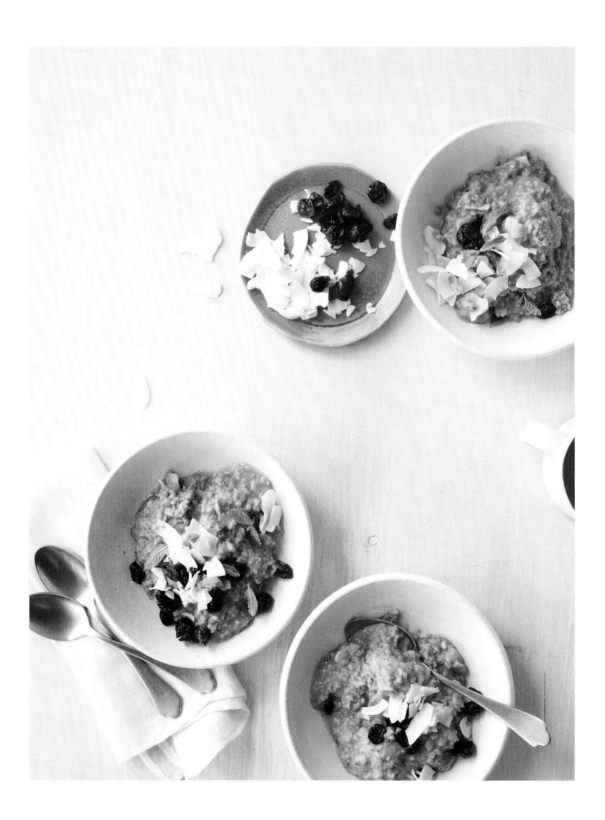

pink energy porridge

Talk about a detoxifier: cranberries contain certain antioxidants that are helpful in preventing and treating pesky urinary tract infections, as well as boosting immunity as they quell inflammation. This is a delicious porridge to eat, midmorning or midafternoon, for an energy-enhancing, cleansing boost.

1 cup cranberries (frozen are okay)

1 cup filtered water

1½ cups coconut milk

1 tablespoon coconut oil

2 tablespoons coconut flakes

1 cup steel-cut oats

Pinch of sea salt

2 tablespoons maple syrup or coconut nectar, or to taste

1. In a blender or food processor, blend the cranberries, filtered water, and coconut milk until smooth, about 20 seconds.

2. In a medium saucepan, melt the coconut oil over low heat. Add the coconut flakes and cook, stirring and toasting them slightly, for about 2 minutes. Add the cranberry mixture, oats, sea salt, and maple syrup. Raise the heat to medium and bring the mixture to a boil, then quickly reduce the heat to medium-low and cook, uncovered, until thick and creamy, about 20 minutes. Serve immediately.

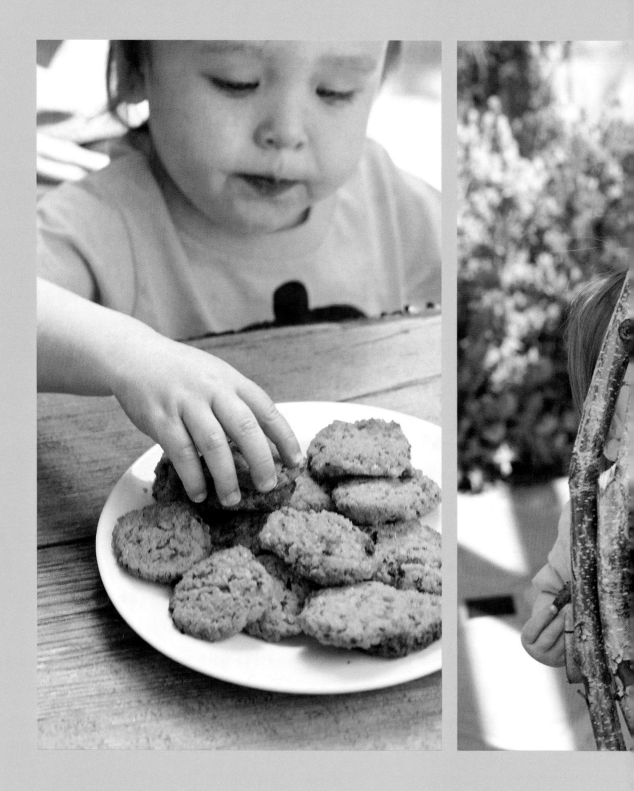

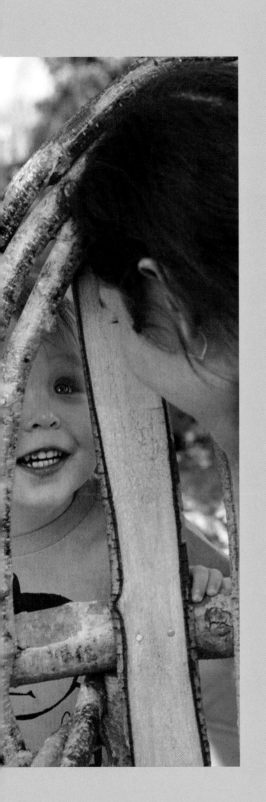

kids' corner

It's an amazing gift to give your children a healthier start by introducing them to healthy recipes. Though they may squirm and toss it from their high chair (like Bubby sometimes!) or, if they are older, plain clam up their mouths and refuse to eat, the very act of offering is love itself. And surveys have found that you may have to offer your child a new food fifteen times or more before they (hopefully) accept it, so keep offering.

These dishes are all delicious, and they are suitable not only for children but also for adults. In fact, I eat and serve all of these recipes to my older children, aka adult friends and family members.

And please don't forget the Glowing Green Smoothie (aka GGS; page 99), which is *the* recipe to share with your young ones to supply them with tons of vitamins, fiber, minerals, and more—it's an incredible practice to get them into as soon as possible! It was Bubby's first food beyond breast milk, and he calls for "GG!" every day (at least at the time of this writing—fingers crossed it continues!). Start them on it early, and they won't yet think green is weird. Or, if they are older or start to develop that "weird" idea, throw in an extra banana, or try making some of the other recipes in the Smoothies chapter or on my website. We can only do our best. Parenting and our kids' diets, just like everything else in life, are going to be perfectly imperfect.

i love you flatbread pizza

MAKES 4 SMALL INDIVIDUAL PIZZAS (ABOUT 6 INCHES IN DIAMETER)

These delicious, healthy pizzas are great for you and the whole fam! The base is the farinata recipe from the Entrées chapter, which is full of protein and minerals such as iron, while being gluten-free. A delicious red sauce and vegan cheese top it off for a yummy, toasty, thin-crust pizza that everyone will request over and over for home-cooked pizza night!

Farinata (page 208)

½ cup Easy Red Sauce (page 185)

1 cup vegan cheese (optional)

½ cup torn fresh basil leaves, for topping (optional)

Dried oregano, for topping

1. Preheat the oven to 350°F.

2. Follow the instructions on page 208 to make the farinata mixture and cook the 4 rounds. Place the farinata rounds on a baking sheet.

3. Spread 2 tablespoons of the red sauce and ¼ cup of the vegan cheese (if using) on each farinata. Bake for about 20 minutes, or until the vegan cheese melts and the crust crisps.

4. Top with the fresh basil (if using) and some dried oregano before serving.

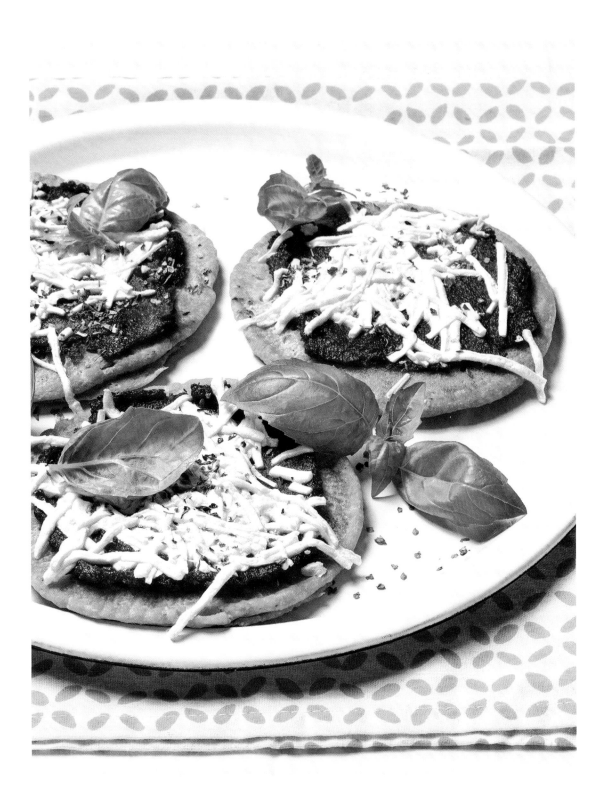

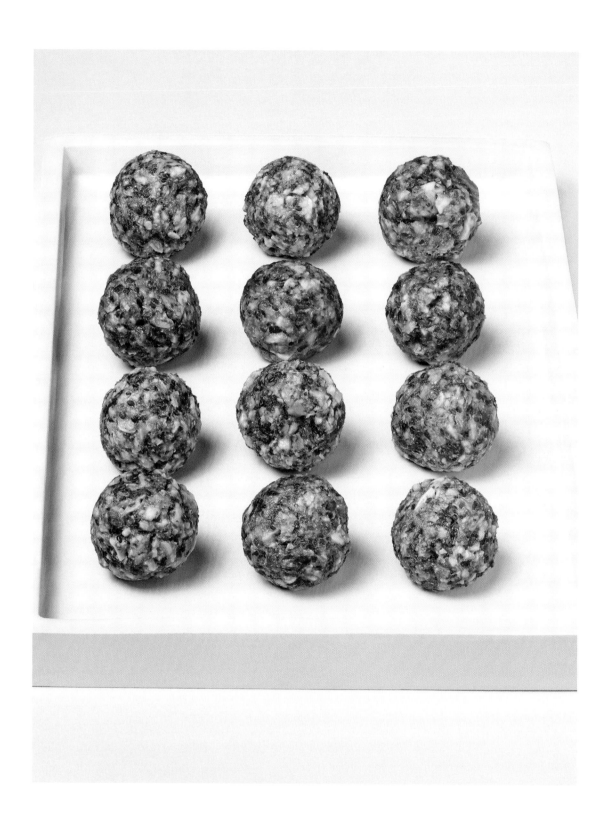

superhero spinach balls

MAKES ABOUT 24 BALLS (1 TO 1¼ INCHES IN DIAMETER)

These delicious bite-size balls supply your little ones' precious bodies with protein, healthy fats (including omega-3 fats), vitamin E, zinc, magnesium, antioxidants, and fiber. If you can get your kids to try them (despite their greenish, spinach-induced hue), I think they will be very surprised at how yummy they are!

1 tablespoon Chia Gel (page 104)

3 cups fresh spinach, well washed and dried

1 cup raw unsalted cashews

½ cup raw unsalted almonds

3 tablespoons olive oil

½ teaspoon sea salt

1 tablespoon nutritional yeast

2 tablespoons garbanzo bean (chickpea) flour

1. Preheat the oven to 350°F and line a baking sheet with parchment paper.

2. In a food processor, combine all the ingredients and pulse until the nuts are slightly ground.

3. Scoop about 2 teaspoons of the spinach mixture from the food processor bowl, shape it into a ball, and place it on the prepared baking sheet (moistening your hands makes it much easier to form the balls). Repeat with the remaining spinach mixture, making sure to leave a few inches between the balls on the baking sheet.

4. Bake for 18 to 20 minutes, until the bottoms of the spinach balls have browned.

5. Remove the baking sheet from the oven and allow it to cool 5 to 10 minutes on a wire cooling rack before removing the spinach balls with a spatula. Eat while warm, or cover and refrigerate for up to 1 week (reheat before serving).

super-yum cheesy cauli tots

MAKES ABOUT 18 BITE-SIZE TOTS

Regular Tater Tots are deep-fried and loaded with sodium. Ugh. The toxicity buildup that goes along with fried foods does no one's body any good, especially your little one's, so this recipe is a great alternative. Plus, these truly are delicious, especially with the inclusion of the vegan Cheddar cheese, which is not totally "perfect," as it is processed and sometimes contains vegetable oil, yet it is super-kid-friendly. And the benefits of eating this recipe are very strong; the tots supply B vitamins, protein, potassium, and vitamin K.

1 tablespoon coconut oil, plus more for greasing

½ large head cauliflower (about 1 pound), cored and coarsely chopped

½ cup vegan Cheddar cheese

2 tablespoons nutritional yeast

2 tablespoons almond flour

¼ teaspoon sea salt

Freshly ground black pepper to taste

2 tablespoons garbanzo bean (chickpea) flour

1. Preheat the oven to 375°F. Grease a baking sheet with coconut oil.

2. In a skillet, melt the 1 tablespoon coconut oil over medium heat. Add the cauliflower and sauté just until it softens, 3 to 4 minutes. Transfer the cauliflower to a food processor and pulse just until it is broken down but still a bit chunky (and not mushy!).

3. In a bowl, combine the chopped cauliflower with the vegan cheese, nutritional yeast, almond flour, sea salt, and pepper. Stir until the ingredients are well combined. Add the garbanzo bean flour and stir until combined.

4. Using a measuring spoon, scoop out a rounded tablespoonful of the mixture and place it on the prepared baking sheet; repeat with the remaining mixture. Bake for 25 to 30 minutes, or until the tots are nicely browned.

banana oatmeal 'n raisin snacks

These easy-to-make energizing bites are perfect for car rides, snacks, packed lunches, and more!

Coconut oil, for greasing

2 large ripe bananas

2 tablespoons almond milk

1 cup quick-cooking oats

½ cup raisins

¼ teaspoon ground cinnamon

1. Preheat the oven to 350°F. Grease a baking sheet with coconut oil.

2. In a bowl, mash the bananas and stir in the almond milk, oats, raisins, and cinnamon. Spoon about 2 tablespoons onto the prepared baking sheet so the round is about 3 inches across. Repeat with the remaining mixture. Bake for 15 minutes, or until the tops are lightly browned.

happy chick chicken-less nuggets

SERVES 4 TO 6;
MAKES 18 NUGGETS

Regular chicken nuggets are not a very happy food, unfortunately. Fast-food chicken nuggets, for instance, can contain over thirty different ingredients, including TBHQ, or tertiary butylhydroquinone, a petroleum-based preservative also used in varnishes and lacquers, which has been shown to cause DNA damage. While I go could on and on about other ingredients and their detrimental effects, it would fill this entire book, so let's just leave it with the fact that there are *many* reasons to avoid commercial chicken nuggets.

No worries, though, as this recipe is delicious for all, nontoxic, and full of protein and other nutrients. Try making a double batch so you can freeze some, ready to thaw out and reheat for your kids' next nuggets cravings!

6 pieces gluten-free bread

patties

1½ cups drained canned artichoke hearts

1½ cups cooked chickpeas, drained and rinsed

¼ cup diced onion

½ cup organic polenta

2 teaspoons red wine vinegar

½ teaspoon sea salt, or to taste

1 cup coconut milk

¼ cup garbanzo bean (chickpea) flour

Freshly ground black pepper to taste

Coconut oil, for greasing

coating

¼ cup organic polenta

1 teaspoon paprika

¼ teaspoon sea salt

Freshly ground black pepper to taste

Radiance Carrot Ketchup (page 217)

1. Preheat the oven to 375°F.

2. Place the gluten-free bread slices on a baking sheet and bake until toasted, about 12 minutes. Remove from the oven and let cool, then process into fine crumbs in a food processor or blender. Set to the side.

3. Make the patties: In a food processor, pulse the artichoke hearts until coarsely chopped. Add the chickpeas, onion, ½ cup of the bread crumbs, the polenta, red wine vinegar, sea salt, coconut milk, and garbanzo bean flour, and mix until well combined. Avoid overprocessing, or the mixture may become mushy! Season with more sea salt, if desired, and with pepper and transfer to an airtight container. Refrigerate for at least 30 minutes, or up to a day.

4. If necessary, preheat the oven again to 375°F. Grease a baking sheet with coconut oil.

5. Make the coating: In a bowl, combine ¼ cup of the bread crumbs with the polenta, paprika, sea salt, and pepper, and stir well.

6. Remove the patty mixture from the refrigerator and using about ¼ cup of the mixture at a time, shape it into 18 nuggets. Tip the nuggets one at a time into the coating mixture, gently flipping them so that both sides get coated. Place the nuggets on the prepared baking sheet and bake for 20 to 22 minutes, until they turn golden brown. Serve with carrot ketchup.

noodles
with sage-pumpkin sauce

SERVES 4

This is a great, all-veggie dish that is creamy and decadent—sans dairy of any kind! It's great for adult cream lovers and kids alike. You can source a veggie spiralizer pretty inexpensively at a home-goods store or online, or simply julienne the zucchini into long, thin noodle shapes.

sage-pumpkin sauce

2 cups pumpkin puree (or 1 [15-ounce] carton, which is close enough to 2 cups)

⅓ cup coconut milk

¼ cup nutritional yeast

2 tablespoons coarsely chopped fresh sage leaves

½ teaspoon sea salt

Freshly ground black pepper to taste

3 medium zucchini, processed in a spiralizer or peeled and julienned (see Note)

2 tablespoons minced fresh parsley, for topping

1. Make the sage-pumpkin sauce: Process the pumpkin puree, coconut milk, nutritional yeast, sage, sea salt, and pepper in a food processor or blender until smooth.

2. Transfer the sauce to a saucepan and warm it gently over low heat until heated through.

3. In a serving bowl, toss the zucchini spirals with the warm sauce. Top with the parsley and serve.

note:
For a heartier dish (and for kids who really love "real" spaghetti!), substitute 12 ounces of gluten-free pasta, cooking according to the package instructions, for the zucchini.

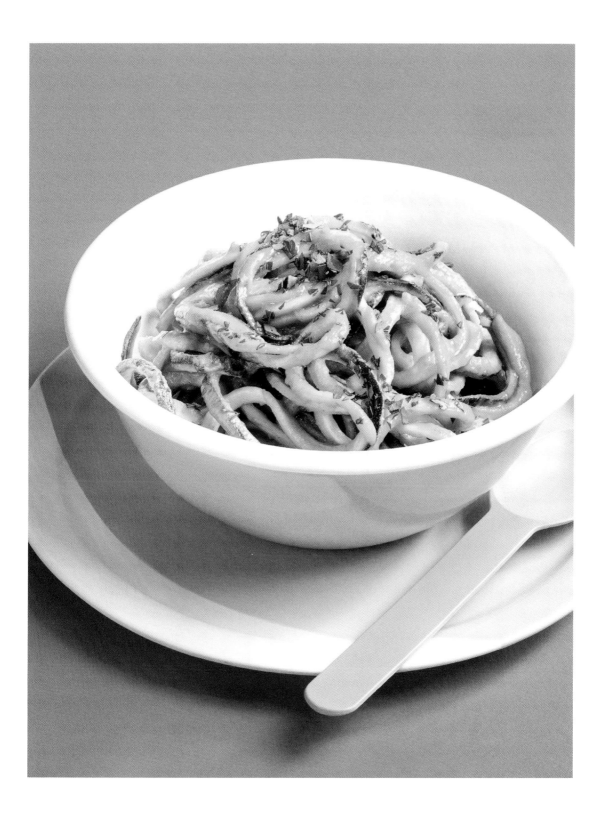

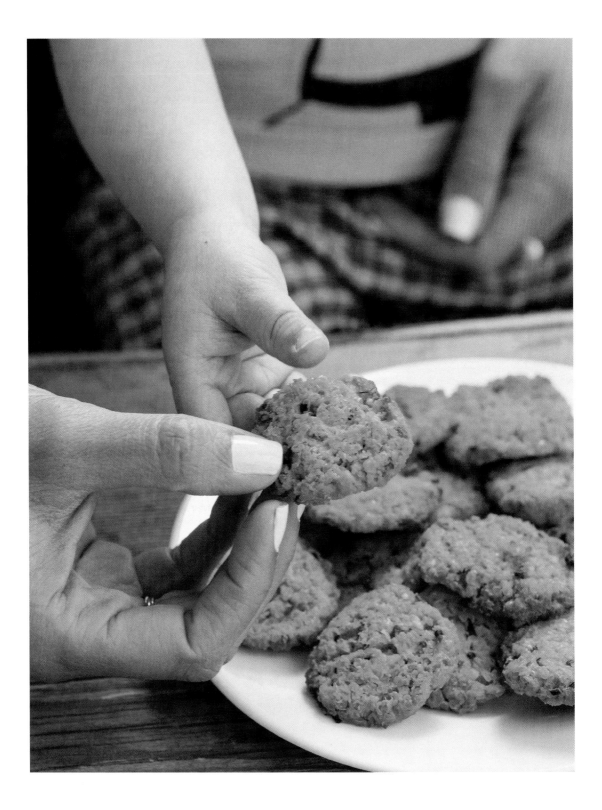

bubby's burgers

MAKES ABOUT 25 MINIATURE BURGERS (ABOUT 2 INCHES IN DIAMETER)

When Bubby was seven weeks old, I traveled to New York City for a press tour for *Radical Beauty*, a book I coauthored with Deepak Chopra. Bubby, of course, came along (often sleeping or nursing on me during my meetings), and we have been traveling the world together ever since.

He was still exclusively nursing then, and that continued for seven months. As he got older, we started adding Glowing Green Smoothies and steamed veggies to his diet. Eventually we introduced these little burgers, which are an incredible travel food. They are great not only for airports and planes but also to take on picnics, to the park, and while running around on errands.

These burgers are high in protein; minerals like iron, folate, and magnesium; vitamins A and C; B vitamins; and many other nutrients. They are flavorful without using any salt. Of course, you can adjust the seasonings for you or your child, but I love that Bubby was used to turmeric and cumin from the start, and he remains open to a wide variety of ethnic and new foods. Try them for yourself and for your little ones!

(RECIPE CONTINUES)

3 medium sweet potatoes (about 1 pound total)

¾ cup quinoa, soaked overnight, rinsed well, and drained

1 tablespoon coconut oil, plus more for greasing (optional)

½ cup small-diced carrots

½ cup small-diced unpeeled zucchini

1 tablespoon ground cumin

1 teaspoon ground turmeric

⅓ cup garbanzo bean (chickpea) flour

1. Bring a pot of water to a boil, add the sweet potatoes, and cook for 25 minutes, or until softened. When the sweet potatoes are done, drain, rinse them with cold water, and peel the skins off.

2. Meanwhile, bring 2½ cups of water to a boil in another pot. Reduce it to a simmer, add the quinoa, and cook for 12 to 14 minutes, until the quinoa is cooked through. Drain off any extra water, and transfer the cooked quinoa to a large mixing bowl.

3. Preheat the oven to 375°F. Grease a baking sheet with coconut oil or use a nonstick baking sheet.

4. Add the carrots and zucchini to the quinoa, along with the cumin and turmeric, and stir to combine.

5. In another bowl and using a fork, mash the sweet potato, 1 tablespoon coconut oil, and garbanzo bean flour. Add this into the quinoa mixture, and mix well to combine.

6. Form miniature "burgers," about 2 inches in diameter, and place them on the prepared (or nonstick) baking sheet. Bake for about 20 minutes on one side, then flip and bake for 10 minutes on the second side, or until they are cooked through to your liking. You can serve several at a time to your little one (and broken down even smaller for little little ones).

protein meat-less balls

MAKES ABOUT 18 BALLS (ABOUT 2 INCHES IN DIAMETER)

This hearty and delicious quinoa-based meatball replacement is full of protein and nutrition, without any processed ground meat. Make them for yourself and your loved ones, knowing you are giving the incredible gift of supporting the health of their bodies and wellness all around!

½ cup quinoa, soaked overnight, rinsed well, and drained

Coconut oil, for greasing

1 tablespoon tamari

¼ teaspoon dried basil

¼ teaspoon dried oregano

¼ teaspoon dried rosemary

½ cup finely chopped cremini mushrooms

½ packed cup finely chopped baby spinach leaves

Juice of ½ lemon

3 tablespoons quick-cooking oats

3 tablespoons garbanzo bean (chickpea) flour

Sea salt and freshly ground black pepper to taste

1. Place the rinsed quinoa into a pot with 1 cup of water. Bring to a boil, reduce the heat, and then simmer, letting it cook all the way down, about 15 minutes. Cool for 10 minutes.

2. Meanwhile, preheat the oven to 350°F. Grease a baking sheet with coconut oil.

3. In a food processor, combine the cooled quinoa, tamari, basil, oregano, rosemary, mushrooms, spinach, lemon juice, oats, and garbanzo bean flour, and process until mixed but still a bit chunky. Season with sea salt and pepper.

4. Scoop out about 2 tablespoons of the quinoa mixture, roll it into a ball, and place it on the prepared baking sheet; repeat with the remaining mixture until 18 equal-size balls are formed, leaving a few inches between them on the baking sheet. Bake for 12 minutes, or until slightly browned. Eat warm, or cover and refrigerate for up to 1 week (reheat before serving).

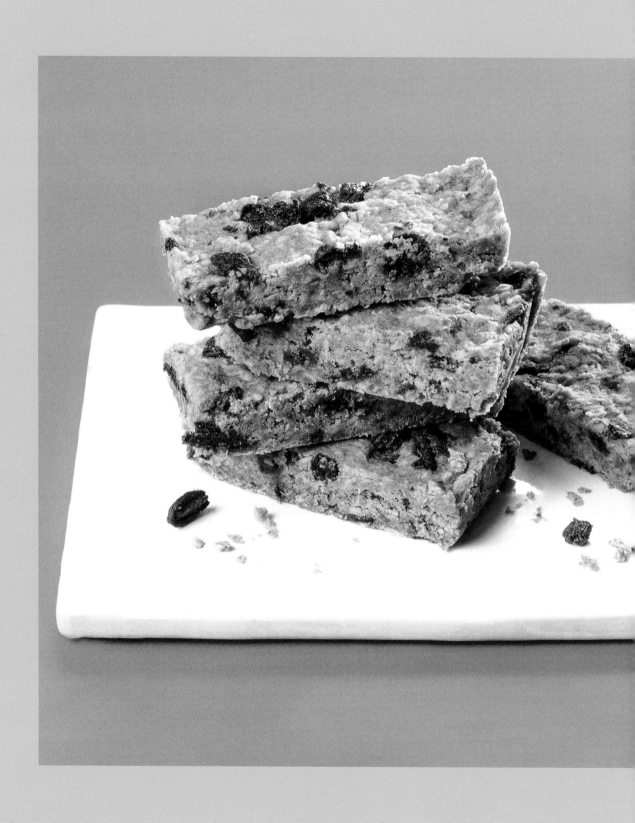

desserts and bars

We all need some sweetness in our lives! After all, life is the mix of all tastes—rich, bitter, sour, pungent, astringent—and definitely also sweet for balance. As you'll see in the following recipes, however, we use healthier sweeteners, such as coconut nectar and coconut sugar, which are low glycemic and low in fructose and contain some minerals; dates, a natural fruit high in calcium and iron that promotes good digestion, are another sweet option. All recipes are free of refined or artificial sweeteners, dairy, gluten, and eggs, and are properly food combined (see page 84 for more info).

Bars are a wonderful way to get a delicious, treat-like food that is still healthy—and that you can pick up and eat. There are zillions of commercial bars out there, yet most of them have processed ingredients, vegetable oils, preservatives, and other yucky components; are improperly food combined; and so on. Making any one of the amazing bars in this section is an incredible way to nurture and rejuvenate yourself, which you absolutely deserve!

goji berry soothe bars

MAKES 12 BARS

Goji berries, which hail from Asia, are one of the most amazing foods in the world to support our vitality and true beauty.

Gojis are rich in antioxidants, which protect our bodies from inflammation and fortify our immunity. They also provide a good source of protein; one serving contains four grams of protein and eighteen different amino acids, as well as more than twenty other trace minerals (including zinc and iron), not to mention vitamins C and A. Gojis can help cleanse and support your liver as well.

These bars contain dried goji berries, which combine well with the other ingredients. The bars come out slightly dry and crumbly, and make a wonderful snack to take on the go or to make for picnics, your kids' lunches, or afternoon treats at the office.

1 cup coconut oil, melted (see Note on page 258), plus more for greasing

2 cups quick-cooking oats

1 cup KS Gluten-Free Flour Mix (page 252)

1 cup coarsely chopped dried goji berries

1½ teaspoons guar gum

¼ teaspoon sea salt

½ cup coconut nectar

1. Preheat the oven to 300°F. Grease a 9 × 9-inch glass baking dish with coconut oil.

2. In a large bowl, mix together the oats, flour mix, goji berries, guar gum, and sea salt.

3. In a separate bowl, combine the 1 cup of melted coconut oil and the coconut nectar, then stir it into the flour mixture.

4. Press the mixture into the prepared baking dish and bake for 25 minutes, or until light brown. Let cool on a wire rack for about 15 minutes. Cut into 12 bars.

sesame pudding

Sesame seeds support our vitality and true beauty. They provide a good deal of calcium, zinc, and other minerals; protein; B vitamins; and many other nutrients. They are a bone- and hair-strengthening food. Black sesame seeds are traditionally used in Asian desserts such as this one, and I've eaten a version of this dessert at Shima, one of my favorite Japanese restaurants in LA. However, I opt here for white sesame seeds, to achieve a lighter and brighter appearance.

¼ teaspoon sea salt

½ cup white sesame seeds

¼ cup almond flour

½ cup coconut sugar, plus more as needed

1 teaspoon vanilla extract

⅓ cup coconut milk

1 tablespoon arrowroot powder

2 tablespoons coconut shreds, for topping

1. In a medium saucepan, heat 3 cups of water and the sea salt over medium-high heat.

2. Meanwhile, grind the sesame seeds using a coffee or spice grinder. The ground seeds should become a little oily and almost look like a paste after about 1 minute. Add the ground sesame seeds to the hot salted water and reduce the heat to medium, stirring to thoroughly mix the seeds into the water.

3. Add the almond flour to the saucepan and stir.

4. Raise the heat back to medium-high, bringing the sesame-nut water to a boil, then reduce the heat back down to medium. Simmer the mixture for 5 to 8 minutes.

5. With the pudding still sitting over medium heat, add the ½ cup coconut sugar, vanilla, coconut milk, and arrowroot powder. As soon as the arrowroot powder is added, stir continuously until everything is thoroughly mixed. The dessert should thicken within a minute or two.

6. Taste for sweetness, adding a little more coconut sugar, if needed. Serve in small dessert cups or bowls while still warm, topped with the coconut shreds.

note:
Although I prefer this dessert served warm, it's also a nice treat served cold on a warm day. To store, keep it in a covered container in the refrigerator for up to 1 week.

wholesome banana crisp

SERVES 6 TO 8

I love crisps! And one of the few fruits to use in a crisp, when adhering to food-combining principles, is the banana, which is a low-water, slower digesting fruit than, say, a peach or apple. The other thing I am a real stickler about is not baking with spreads that contain vegetable oils, which become rancid at higher temperatures. I always opt for coconut oil, which combines well with the sweetener to ensure a non-coconut taste and still holds its structural integrity at a high temperature in the oven. It's great for our sweet tooth . . . and for our energy and skin!

1 tablespoon
  coconut oil

filling

1¼ cups coconut sugar

⅓ cup tapioca flour

2 tablespoons coconut
  milk

6 ripe bananas, cut into
  1½-inch pieces

topping

1 cup quick-cooking
  oats

½ cup coconut sugar

¼ cup brown rice flour

¼ cup garbanzo bean
  (chickpea) flour

½ teaspoon ground
  nutmeg

½ teaspoon ground
  cinnamon

¾ cup coconut oil,
  melted (see Note on
  page 258)

Vanilla coconut ice
  cream, for serving
  (optional)

1. Preheat the oven to 350°F. Grease an 8-inch square baking dish with the 1 tablespoon coconut oil.

2. Make the filling: In a small bowl, mix together the coconut sugar and tapioca flour, then mash in the coconut milk and bananas, stirring to combine. Pour the filling into the prepared baking dish.

3. Make the topping: In a bowl, mix all the topping ingredients together until thoroughly combined yet still chunky, and spread it evenly over the filling. Bake, uncovered, for about 30 minutes, or until the top is browned and crispy (see Note). Let cool on a wire rack for at least 10 minutes before serving with vanilla coconut ice cream, if desired.

note:
After 30 minutes of baking, the inside of the crisp will be soft while the outside will be drier and harder. I love gooier desserts! It is safe to eat it this way, as this recipe contains no egg or any other type of animal products.

ks gluten-free flour mix

MAKES 3 CUPS

When you're baking gluten-free and vegan, you absolutely *must* have a mix of gluten-free flours for your recipes to work. Trust me, this recipe has come from an incredible amount of trial and error! I've finally discovered that it is so much easier to have a premade gluten-free flour mix handy in the kitchen, rather than trying to portion out individual amounts of each flour or ingredient for every recipe.

It's great to double, triple, or even quadruple this recipe so it's always ready to go whenever you feel like baking some of these yummy desserts!

1 cup tapioca flour

¼ cup brown rice flour

¾ cup garbanzo bean (chickpea) flour

¾ cup sorghum flour

¼ cup teff flour

Place all the ingredients in a gallon-size ziplock bag, seal it, and toss it around to thoroughly combine everything. You can store the flour mix in the refrigerator for up to 6 months or in the freezer for up to 1 year.

raw beauty spirulina bars

This is a fortifying bar that will give you strength, mentally and spiritually—and even for your hair! Spirulina is a natural algae that is incredibly high in protein; it's over 60 percent protein by weight. It is also a great source of antioxidants and B vitamins, as well as vitamins A, K_1, and K_2. It is rich in minerals such as iron, manganese, and chromium, and phytonutrients including carotenoids, gamma linolenic acid (GLA), superoxide dismutase (SOD), and phycocyanin. Here's an amazing fact: spirulina contains a whopping 2,800 percent more beta-carotene than carrots.

Here's the thing, though: spirulina tastes like, well, algae. Therefore, it is essential to balance spirulina with other ingredients in the right way to make sure it is yummy so that you keep enjoying the benefits. And this recipe does just that.

1 cup raw unsalted cashews

¼ cup hempseeds

1 tablespoon cacao powder

¾ teaspoon spirulina

⅛ teaspoon sea salt

¼ teaspoon peeled and minced fresh ginger

9 dates, pitted

Coconut oil, for greasing

1. In a food processor, combine the cashews, hempseeds, cacao power, spirulina, sea salt, and ginger; pulse to mix well. Add the dates and process until the mixture is evenly chopped.

2. Grease a 9 × 9-inch glass baking dish with coconut oil. Press the mixture into the dish so it forms an even layer. Cover the dish with plastic wrap, and refrigerate for 30 to 45 minutes. To serve, cut into bars using a clean knife that you've run under hot water.

lemon and orange zest bars

**MAKES 16 SMALL
SQUARES**

These bars are incredibly bright and zesty, and they will power you for the day ahead! They're a delicious snack for an afternoon (or pretty much anytime) pick-me-up—get ready for a sweet, citrusy blast.

1¼ cups coconut oil, melted (see Note on page 258), plus more for greasing

2 cups quick-cooking oats

1 cup KS Gluten-Free Flour Mix (page 252)

½ teaspoon freshly grated lemon zest

3 tablespoons fresh lemon juice

1 tablespoon grated orange zest

1½ teaspoons guar gum

¼ teaspoon sea salt

¾ cup coconut nectar

1. Preheat the oven to 300°F. Grease a 9 × 9-inch glass baking dish with coconut oil. Set to the side.

2. In a large bowl, mix together the oats, flour mix, lemon zest, lemon juice, orange zest, guar gum, and sea salt.

3. In a separate bowl, combine the 1¼ cups coconut oil and the coconut nectar, then stir it into the flour mixture.

4. Press the mixture into the prepared baking dish and bake for 25 minutes, or until light brown. Let cool for about 15 minutes on a wire rack, then cut into bars. Enjoy immediately, or cover and refrigerate for up to 1 week.

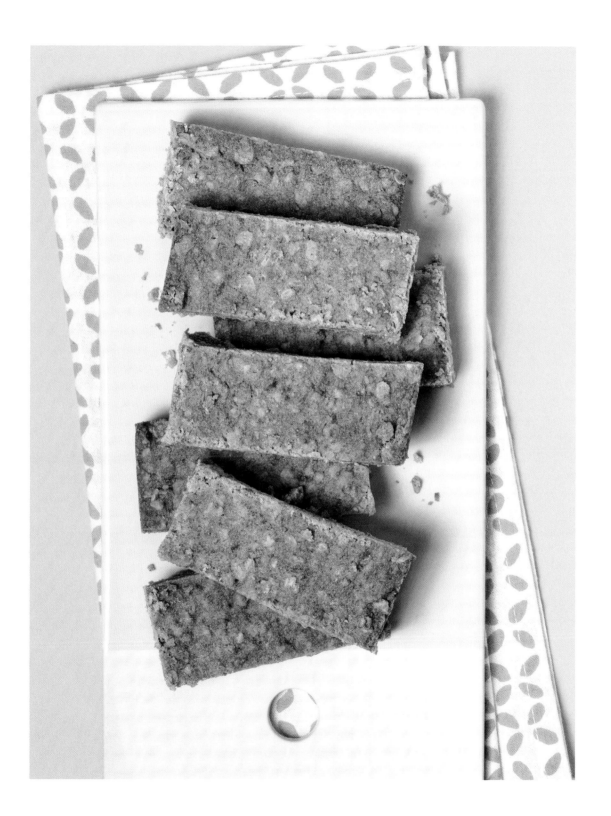

figalicious bars

MAKE 20 SMALL BARS

Figs are a wonderful cleansing, detoxifying food that helps flush out your system. They also contain B vitamins and minerals such as iron, calcium, and potassium.

2 cups quick-cooking oats

1 cup KS Gluten-Free Flour Mix (page 252)

1 teaspoon ground cinnamon

¼ cup coconut sugar

1 teaspoon guar gum

¼ teaspoon sea salt

½ cup coconut oil, melted (see Note on page 258)

1 teaspoon vanilla extract

¼ cup coconut nectar

12 fresh Calimyrna figs, destemmed and coarsely chopped

1. Preheat the oven to 300°F. Line a 9 × 9-inch glass baking dish with parchment paper, letting it hang over the sides.

2. In a large bowl, mix together the oats, flour, cinnamon, coconut sugar, guar gum, and sea salt.

3. In a separate bowl, combine the coconut oil, vanilla, and coconut nectar, then stir it into the flour mixture. Mix in the fig chunks.

4. Press the mixture into the prepared baking dish and bake for 25 minutes, or until light brown. Let cool for about 15 minutes on a wire rack, then cut into bars. Enjoy immediately, or cover the dish and refrigerate for up to 1 week.

raw sunshine energy bars

MAKES ABOUT 8 BARS

Seeds are amazing fortifying foods, protecting our vitality and keeping us strong for the ups and downs of our daily journeys. Sunflower and pumpkin seeds supply zinc, magnesium, copper, B vitamins, healthy fats, and vitamin E.

½ cup sunflower seeds

⅓ cup pumpkin seeds

1 teaspoon ground
   cinnamon

¼ teaspoon ground
   cardamom

¼ teaspoon ground
   nutmeg

⅛ teaspoon sea salt

14 Medjool dates, pitted

1. In a food processor, combine all the ingredients except for the dates; pulse to mix well. Add the dates and process until the mixture is evenly chopped.

2. Press the mixture into a 9 × 9-inch glass baking dish, cover with plastic wrap, and place in the fridge for 30 to 45 minutes. To serve, cut it into bars using a clean knife that you've run under hot water.

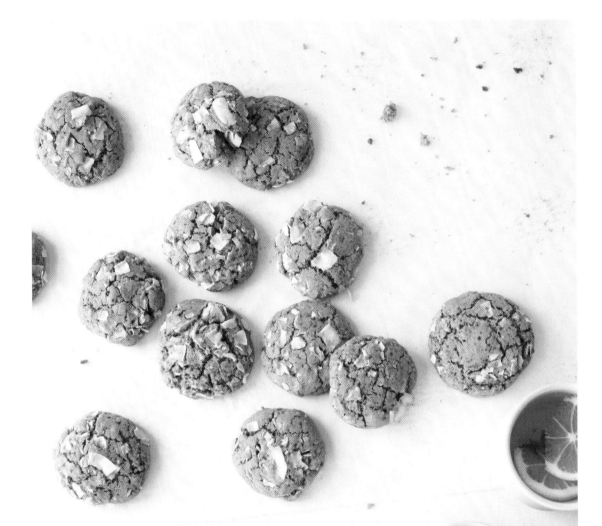
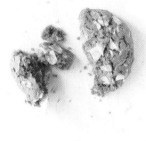
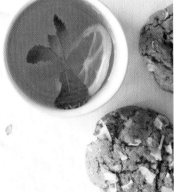

note:

From a baking standpoint, what is incredibly important about coconut oil is that it has a high smoke point and does not become denatured at higher temperatures. That is why it is the only oil that I bake with! I don't recommend baking with vegetable oil–containing spreads that can become rancid at higher temperatures.

coconut wow cookies

There are currently over 1,500 studies on the benefits of coconut oil. As it is sent to your liver to be processed, coconut oil helps increase your metabolism and provides longer sustained energy. A study published in the journal *Antimicrobial Agents and Chemotherapy* found the capric acid and lauric acid in coconut oil made for an effective natural treatment for *Candida albicans* and yeast infections.

For coconut lovers out there, these delicious cookies really highlight the earthy coconut flavor with the inclusion of the coconut flakes.

2 cups KS Gluten-Free Flour Mix (page 252)

½ teaspoon baking soda

½ teaspoon guar gum

½ cup coconut sugar

¼ teaspoon sea salt

¼ cup coconut oil, melted (see Note)

¼ cup coconut nectar

1 teaspoon vanilla extract

⅓ cup almond milk

1 cup coconut flakes

1. Preheat the oven to 325°F. Line a baking sheet with parchment paper. Set to the side.

2. In a large bowl, whisk together the flour mix, baking soda, guar gum, coconut sugar, and sea salt. Make a well in the middle.

3. In a separate bowl, combine the melted coconut oil, coconut nectar, vanilla, and almond milk, and stir well. Pour the liquid into the well in the flour mixture. Stir in the coconut flakes.

4. Shape about 1 tablespoon of the mixture into a ball and place it on the parchment-lined baking sheet. Gently flatten it with the palm of your hand so it pushes outward into a flat cookie shape. Continue until all the dough is formed into cookies, being sure to place them a few inches apart.

5. Bake the cookies for 13 to 14 minutes, until they are golden brown. Transfer them from the baking sheet to a wire rack and let cool for at least 15 minutes before serving.

mint-chocolate lover's brownies

MAKES 16 BROWNIES

The fresh mint in this recipe is bright tasting and even helps promote digestion. These are soft and mushy and gooey, versus the denser texture of some brownies. Of course, if you prefer the latter, you can simply bake them a bit longer!

½ cup coconut oil, melted (see Note on page 258), plus more for greasing

1½ cups KS Gluten-Free Flour Mix (page 252)

½ cup cacao powder

¾ teaspoon baking powder

⅓ cup finely minced fresh mint leaves

¼ teaspoon baking soda

¼ teaspoon guar gum

¼ teaspoon sea salt

¾ cup coconut sugar

¾ cup almond milk

⅓ cup coconut nectar

1 teaspoon vanilla extract

¼ teaspoon peppermint flavor

1. Preheat the oven to 325°F. Grease an 8 × 8-inch baking dish with coconut oil.

2. In a large bowl, whisk together the flour mix, cacao, baking powder, mint, baking soda, guar gum, sea salt, and coconut sugar. Make a well in the middle.

3. In a separate bowl, combine the ½ cup coconut oil with the almond milk, coconut nectar, vanilla, and peppermint flavor and stir well. Add this to the well in the flour mixture and stir.

4. Scrape the mixture into the prepared baking dish. Bake for 16 to 17 minutes. Let the pan cool on a wire rack for at least 20 minutes (see Note). Cut into 16 brownies using a clean knife that you've run under hot water.

note:
It is helpful to place the whole pan in the freezer for 20 minutes to harden the brownies so they are easier to cut.

dark chocolate delish tart

MAKES ONE 9-INCH
TART; SERVES 12

Sometimes we just need a "food hug" to help lift us up. In Part I we discussed working on cleansing the deeper roots of negative feelings, but occasionally we need an immediate Band-Aid. And that is okay, too. Cacao is perfect for this, as it is helps boost our moods. It contains anandamide, a neurotransmitter referred to as the "bliss molecule." It also has anti-inflammatory properties, antioxidants, and anthocyanins to help protect our cells, preserve our nervous systems, and keep us radiant. Get ready for a big "food hug" with this rich tart. (Note: This tart is what Bubby and I are noshing on on page 64.)

crust

2 cups almond flour

½ cup coconut oil, melted (see Note on page 258)

12 pitted Medjool dates, chopped

filling

2 cups cacao powder

1 cup coconut nectar or maple syrup

1 cup coconut sugar

1 cup coconut oil, melted

1. Make the crust: In a food processor, process all the crust ingredients until well combined. Press the dough evenly into a 9-inch tart pan with a removable bottom. Cover with plastic wrap and chill in the fridge while preparing the filling.

2. Make the filling: In the food processor or a blender, blend all the filling ingredients until smooth. Pour the filling into the chilled tart crust. Cover with plastic wrap and set in the refrigerator for at least 3 hours before slicing and serving.

fudgy clean blonde brownies

MAKES 16 BROWNIES

Vegan, gluten-free, and properly food combined baking is no easy feat! I have to say that I am very happy with how delicious this recipe is. When I was testing this, I ate almost a third of the container myself in one sitting! Like the Mint-Chocolate Lover's Brownies (page 260), these brownies come out supersoft and fudgy. As I suggest in the Note, throwing them in the freezer for 20 minutes or so makes them easier to cut. I hope you love them as much as I do!

¼ cup coconut oil, melted (see Note on page 258), plus more for greasing

2 cups KS Gluten-Free Flour Mix (page 252)

¾ teaspoon baking powder

¼ teaspoon ground coriander

¼ teaspoon ground cardamom

¼ teaspoon baking soda

¼ teaspoon guar gum

¼ teaspoon sea salt

½ cup coconut sugar

⅓ cup almond milk

¼ cup coconut nectar

2 teaspoons vanilla extract

¾ cup plus ⅓ cup organic vegan dark chocolate chips

1. Preheat the oven to 325°F. Grease an 8 × 8-inch baking dish with coconut oil.

2. In a large bowl, whisk together the flour mix, baking powder, coriander, cardamom, baking soda, guar gum, sea salt, and coconut sugar. Make a well in the middle.

3. In a separate bowl, combine the almond milk, ¼ cup coconut oil, coconut nectar, and vanilla and mix thoroughly. Stir into the well in the flour mixture until well combined though slightly lumpy. Stir in the ¾ cup chocolate chips.

4. Scrape the mixture into the prepared baking dish. Sprinkle the remaining ⅓ cup chocolate chips on top. Bake for 15 to 16 minutes, until the top turns a light golden brown. Let cool on a wire rack for at least 20 minutes (see Note). Cut into 16 brownies using a clean knife that you have run under hot water.

note:

I highly recommend placing the pan in the freezer for at least 20 minutes to help harden the brownies before cutting. They won't be warm, but they will be a more solid, gooey, fudgy deliciousness that you can cut much more easily.

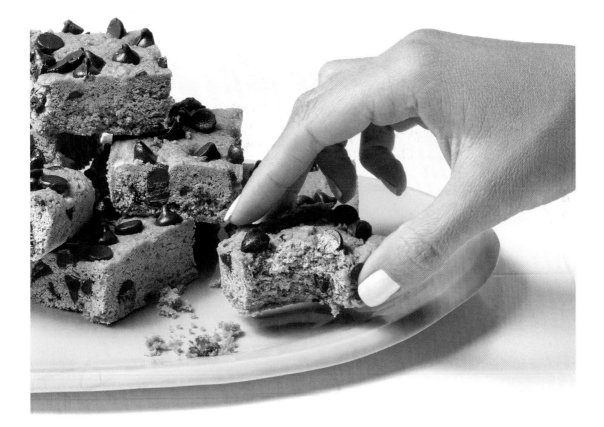

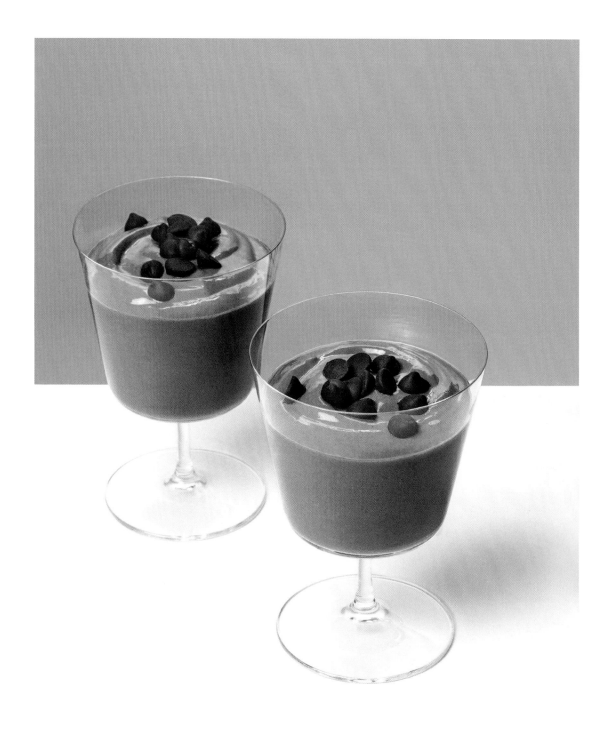

chocolate acai mousse

I've traditionally used nut milks, nuts and seeds, and avocados to make mousse, fudge, and other desserts, yet I am new to using organic, non-GMO tofu for them. I have to say that it works pretty darn well! It creates a substantial base. As I state on page 85, organic soy is okay to rotate into our diets (assuming no soy allergy). The antioxidant-rich acai berry also contains healthy omega fats and is naturally sugar-free, making it one of our exceptions to the food-combining rule regarding fruit.

3 tablespoons cacao powder

⅓ cup coconut sugar

1 tablespoon coconut nectar or maple syrup

1 teaspoon vanilla extract

1 (14-ounce) container organic, non-GMO extra-firm tofu

2 (100-gram) packets unsweetened acai (see page 87)

¼ cup organic vegan dark chocolate chips, for topping

1. In a food processor, combine all the ingredients except the dark chocolate chips and pulse until smooth.

2. Spoon the mixture evenly into four 6-ounce ramekins. Top with the dark chocolate chips. Cover with plastic wrap and chill for at least 20 minutes. Be sure to enjoy it all within 3 days!

double chocolate chip and oatmeal cookies

MAKES 14 COOKIES

These are simple to make, have a good texture that binds nicely, and supply a dense chocolate taste with no gluten or white sugar. How can you go wrong? Be sure to source cacao over cocoa for more nutritional value (swapping an extra *a* over an *o* does make a big difference!).

1 cup KS Gluten-Free Flour Mix (page 252)

½ cup cacao powder

½ teaspoon baking soda

½ teaspoon guar gum

¼ cup coconut oil, melted

¼ cup coconut nectar

½ cup coconut sugar

2 teaspoons vanilla extract

½ teaspoon stevia powder

1¼ cups quick-cooking oats

¾ cup organic vegan chocolate chips

1. Preheat the oven to 325°F. Line a 15 × 13-inch baking sheet with parchment paper.

2. In a large bowl, whisk together the flour mix, cacao, baking soda, and guar gum. Make a well in the middle.

3. In a separate bowl, mix together the coconut oil, coconut nectar, coconut sugar, vanilla, and stevia. Pour the liquid into the well in the flour mixture, along with ½ cup of water, the oats, and the chocolate chips. Stir until all the liquid is absorbed.

4. Shape about 1¼ tablespoons of the dough into a ball and place it on the prepared baking sheet. Gently flatten it with the palm of your hand so it pushes outward into a flat cookie shape. Continue until all the dough is formed into cookies, being sure to place them a few inches apart.

5. Bake for 12 minutes. Let the cookies cool on the baking sheet for a few minutes, then transfer them to a wire cooling rack and let sit for about 10 minutes before serving.

ginger comedown hot chocolate

SERVES 1

Dessert drinks are a great way to satisfy a sweet fix without being too heavy. Because they are liquid, they feel filling and grounding without adding to digestive burden. Ginger is a potent herb that enhances metabolism and digestion, so it's perfect to consume post-meals. With these two ingredients, this is a truly delicious elixir to satisfy as well as nourish you.

1 cup coconut or almond milk

1 (1½-inch) piece of fresh ginger, peeled and thinly sliced

1 tablespoon cacao powder

Dash of ground cinnamon

Pinch of freshly ground black pepper

Coconut sugar to taste

1. In a small saucepan, heat the milk and ginger over high heat and bring to just under a boil. Quickly reduce the heat and simmer for 3 minutes.

2. Stir in the remaining ingredients and serve immediately.

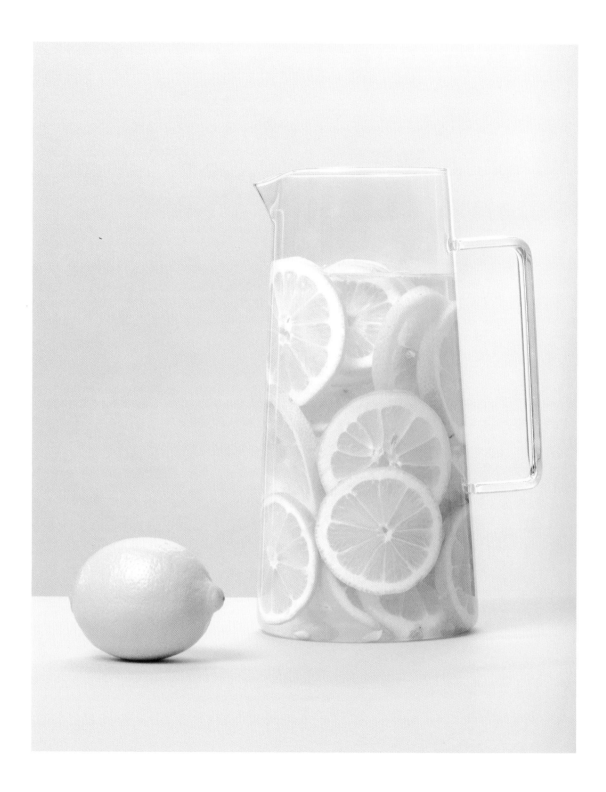

Acknowledgments

The greatest gratitude goes to my incredible friend and editor, Gary Jansen. Gary, thank you so much for helping me organize my ideas, guiding this book to how it is today, believing strongly in me and my work, and on top of all that, simply being a close friend who I love so much. I have the deepest respect for your brilliance and bright, sensitive spirit. You are the best! Thank you, thank you.

And an enormous round of thanks to Aaron Wehner, Diana Baroni, Tammy Blake, Christina Foxley, Brianne Sperber, Patricia Shaw, Jennifer Wang, Marysarah Quinn, Stephanie Huntwork, Ashley Hong, Heather Williamson, and all the other amazing members on the Harmony Penguin Random House team, for your collaboration and belief in me, and for bringing this book out into the world.

Infinite gratitude goes to my Solluna team, especially John Pisani, my long-term business partner. John, thank you for being a rock of support, love, and wisdom, always. I love you back. And thank you to my Goddess team members, especially Katelyn Hughes (aka Earth Mama), for embodying the light, love, and mission in action. And to all the rest of my beloved team. Our sacred circle is so magical.

Huge thank-you to Todd Rubinstein for so generously offering up your beautiful Apple Creek Ranch for our team to camp out and shoot all these photos. Thank you to Diego Saenz for so lovingly and diligently helping me test all these recipes! Thank you to Ylva Erevall, my longtime dear friend and photographer extraordinaire who shot the cover and many of these photos, as well as Victoria Wall Harris, for shooting some of the other great shots that line these pages.

There are not enough words to thank my village. Thank you—sending so much love to you, Dad/Lolo. I am so grateful to you for being such an amazing father, and for us to have this special time together where you get to see EE every day. What a blessing. And Mom, in the spirit world, I feel your love every day and love you more than ever. Thank you, Laura Pringle, dear friend and soul sister who held the space and helped me really connect back with myself, and who also provided some input for this book. You are amazing and I love you! And Tita, for your loving and patient presence, and for maintaining our home during this whole book process and Mom's passing, as well as Auntie and all my dear Mama and other friends. Especially Maki, Esther, Kela, and Ani. And Justin Cava Jones, for inspiring me with your life and teachings. Thank you, Mick, for sharing an amazing part of the journey together, and for being a great co-parent and dad. I love you always.

Last, but not least, infinite gratitude to Bubby, my little angel prince. You are such a powerful, delicious, joyful teacher to me, and I love you beyond words.

We are all part of the One Spirit.
—Paramahansa Yogananda

About the Author

Kimberly Snyder is the founder of Solluna, a holistic lifestyle brand, leader of the #FeelGoodMovement, and the multi-time *New York Times* bestselling author of the Beauty Detox book series and of *Radical Beauty*, cowritten with Deepak Chopra.

An in-demand worldwide speaker, Snyder also hosts the top-rated *Feel Good with Kimberly Snyder* podcast, which airs on the PodcastOne network. In 2018, she opened the Solluna organic juice and smoothie bar at the iconic Four Seasons Hotel in Beverly Hills, Los Angeles.

A certified nutritionist, Snyder has worked with the entertainment industries' top celebrities, including Drew Barrymore, Kerry Washington, Reese Witherspoon, and Channing Tatum, among many others. A highly sought-after lifestyle-and-wellness expert, Snyder has been featured in media outlets that include *Ellen, Today, The Dr. Oz Show,* the *New York Times, Vogue, Vanity Fair,* the *Wall Street Journal, Elle,* and *InStyle*. She is a member of the Wellness Council for Well+Good and was named one of the top "results-oriented nutritionists" by *Vogue*.

Snyder is a member of the Board of Advisors for Visionary Women, a nonprofit organization that supports the empowerment of women. She also works with the Seeds of Hope charity, which focuses on building sustainable vegetable gardens in Los Angeles public schools.

After graduating magna cum laude from Georgetown University, Snyder didn't choose an ordinary path. Instead, she embarked on a three-year solo journey spanning more than fifty countries. This exposed her to a wide range of health-and-beauty modalities, conventional and unconventional teachers, and worldviews from different cultures. This experience inspired her life's journey into wellness.

She continued her studies at various other locations, including the American University of Complementary Medicine, where she completed a four-year Ayurvedic practitioner program.

A passionate practitioner of Kriya Yoga meditation, world adventurer, and mama, Snyder has dedicated her life to inspiring and helping others realize a more joyful life by embracing who they are through all the cycles of their lives.

Paramahansa Yogananda's site (my guru and the meditation I practice): yogananda-srf.org.

Gary's amazing spiritual books and lecture info: garyjansen.com.

Laura's intuitive coaching and workshops: laurapringle.com.

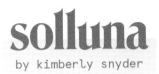

by kimberly snyder

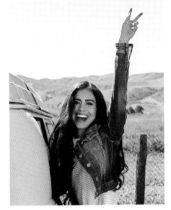

Our mission at Solluna is to help you develop a lifestyle that promotes health, wholeness, self-acceptance, healing, and inclusion for all.

Solluna, a uniting of the sun and moon, means living in harmony with the rhythms of Mother Nature while embracing all the cycles of life—the highs and lows and all the moments in-between.

We are individuals and we are One. As a community, we meet one another where we are in life. Through our messaging, products, practices, and the #FEELGOODMOVEMENT, we are dedicated to empowering you in realizing a more joyful life by embracing yourself and your dreams.

SOLLUNA PRINCIPLES

Unconditional Love
Acceptance and Compassion
Soft and Gentle is Powerful with Clarity
Service to All

Nonjudgment of Self and Others
Everyone's Journey is Unique
Beauty and Appreciation
Oneness

THE #FEELGOODMOVEMENT

FEELING GOOD is *not* about having a picture-perfect life with a flawless body, job, family, and so on. That's all outside stuff. We can have those things and still feel deeply unhappy. So it's not about what we have, but rather finding a level of inner peace in our perfectly imperfect lives.

Yes, we can strive for improvement. Yet at the same time, we can live from a place of understanding that no matter how we look or what we do, we're already whole, complete, and okay as we are.

FEELING GOOD is about accepting our inner compass, which can guide us in making decisions and tuning out the comparisons, overanalyzing, self-doubt, and pretending that causes so much turmoil in our lives.

Sharing our journeys is a powerful way to embrace who we are. Post your story and tag us in your photos, videos, and stories. We want to be there for your highs and lows, and all the moments in-between.

#mysolluna #feelgoodmovement @sollunabyks

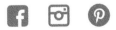

For supplements, skincare, digital programs, and to join our Feel Good Circle and community, go to ♥:

mysolluna.com